FRCR PART 1

MCQs
Radiophysics
Conventional Radiography

Computed Radiography

Digital Radiography

Gamma imaging

MRI

USG

Dr.Nagendra Kumar Sinha
MD (Radio-diagnosis)

TO

MY FATHER

(DWARIKA PRASAD)

WHO TAUGHT ME TO FOLLOW OPEN-ENDED PATH

PREFACE

MCQs is a standard format to assess the conceptual and factual knowledge. FRCR has adopted the same approach ,with each statement to be judged TRUE OR FALSE. In such scenario, either you are correct or chances of being correct or wrong remains 50:50 in case of gauessing . So, one need to be very careful in answering such questions. Only way to get confidence is to solve as many questions as possible .So ,I have tried to present the most comprehensive book of MCQs (radiophysics) on line of the latest syllabus of FRCR. There are about **1200 MCQs (1200 x5 =6500 statements)** covering each and every aspect of syllabus of FRCR including MRI and USG..Each MCQs is followed by answer with relevant explanation with reference. I wish to bring to emphasize that most of MCQs are based on two most important books for FRCR ---1. **4ᵗʰ edition ,1990 reprinted 2010 , Christensen's Physics of Diagnostic radiology and 2.second edition(2008),Farr's Physics for Medical Imaging.**I believe this book will prove to be perfect revision tool for candidate sitting in the FRCR PART 1.This MCQs book will surely be of great help and guidance for those who aspire to clear the exam of FRCR.

Besides,this book will be useful for all those doctors ,residents and technicians who wish to make concept of radiophysics more clear.

Wishing you all the best,

Nagendra Kumar Sinha

E-mail:ngdrkus@yahoo.co.in

Blog:nagendra's radiology blog

CONTENTS

ACKNOWLEDGEMENTS

I am grateful to ALMIGHTY GOD who inspired and gave me strength to write this book.

I am grateful to my teachers,particularly Dr. N K Gogoi and Dr R K Gogoi, who chided me for my ignorance and prodded me towards excellence,

I am grateful to my father late Dwarika Prasad and mother

Smt Kaushalya devi for their constant blessings

I really feel privileged to extend my gratitude to my brother

 Er.S K P Sinha and sister-in law Manjula Rani Renu.

I am grateful to my wife Rina sinha and my son Anmol Kumar Sinha and Rajat Kumar Sinha for sacrifice they made during my engagement .

I am highly indebtebted to my father-in-law R A Roy and

mother –in -law Aruna Roy and sister-in law Anju Roy and Nina Roy .

I am grateful to my colleagues and seniors for their support ,cooperation and suggestions ,to name a few—Dr,Akshay Dharmarha,Dr Naveen Niraj,Dr C L Verma Dr.Pavan Pandey,Dr,Mukesh Verma, Dr.Vidya Nandan, Dr.Jitendra Dahiya,Dr. Bhupender Singh ,Dr.Surendra Singh ,Dr.Suman

Bharati ,Dr.Amit Sinha ,Dr.Bharat ,Dr.Druv Pathak ,Dr,Anil

Shahani ,Dr.P K Jain ,Dr.D K Jha ,Dr.Mukesh Prasad ,

Dr.Mukesh Singh, Dr.Lokesh, Dr.B P Sharma, Dr. Sanjay Gupta, Dr.Manoj Kumar, Dr.Naveen Niraj, Dr.Sanjay Mintoo ,Dr,Rajnish, Dr.Jyotsana Rani Malik Dr.ansari , Dr.lokesh, Dr.Dev, Dr.Sunil Sahdev , Dr.Nidhi , Dr.shittal Dr.Arun ,Dr. Prashant ,Dr. Anand ,

Dr. Anuj Bhatnagar ,Dr.Arun Choudhary,Dr.arun yadav,Dr.Parineeta Hazarika,Dr.Sharaf Alam ,Dr.Ravindra Sharma ,Dr. Shahaj Chopra,Dr.Kirti,Dr. M Mehra,Dr.Permanand

,Dr.Purvey ,Dr.K K Sinha.

I feel great gratitude to Mrs Ranju Vij , Mrs Manju and Mr Ved pal

I am grateful to Facebook and Nagendra's radiology blog fraternity who responded and appreciated the questions

 posted by me during manuscripts preparation.

Special thanks to my friend Sanjay Jayaswal and Asok Kumar who is always with me in all time and everytime.

Last but not the least ,I am indebted to createspace for providing me plateform to publish this book.

Nagendra kumar sinha

CHAPTER 1
Basics Physics

1.True regarding atoms
a. tungsten has a K shell energy of 70 keV
b. tungsten has a L shell energy of 11 keV
c. atomic number of tungsten is 74
d. atomic number of copper is 29
e. copper has a K shell energy of 9 keV

2. True regarding atoms is/are
a. the binding energy of K electrons shells remains same for all elements
b. an electron of an atom can move from K shell to L shell by emission of energy
c. K shell has subsets of slightly different energy energies
d. forbidden transition refers to anability of an L electron in the lowest subshell to move to the K shell
e. The diameter of the atom is about 100,000 times larger than the diameter of its its nucleus

3. True regarding an atom
a. K shell is closest to the nucleus
b. binding force refers to the attractive force between the nucleus and the electron
c .L electron has larger binding force than an an K electron
d. electrons in an atom is in positive energy states
e. the binding energy of the electron refers to energy required to raise its value to zero

4. True regarding photons is/are
a. discrete bundles of energy
b. energy of photons depend on its frequency
c. travels at the speed of light
d. the unit to measure the energy of photons is EV.
e. ionizing radiation'photon energy is =<15 ev

5.True regarding EM radiation is/are
a. propagate through a vaccum
b. different EM radiations have the same velocity
c. the velocity in vaccum is 3x 10^8 meters /sec
d. EM radiations differ only in wavelength
e. no overlap in wavelengths of various EM radiations

6. True statement regarding photon and ionizing radiation is/are
A.Energy of photons in keV =24.2/wavelength(A^0)
b. Plank's constant /frequency of photon give the energy of photons
c. an atom gains an electron on ionisation
d. x ray energies are usually measured in EV
e. gamma rays and x rays and some ultraviolet rays are ionizing radiation.

7. True regarding EM radiation is/are
a. propagate through a vaccum
b. different EM radiations have the same velocity
c. the velocity in vaccum is 3x 10^8

meters /sec

d. EM radiations differ only in wavelength

e. No overlap in wavelengths of various EM radiations

8. Correctly matched SI unit is/are

a. radioactivity—becquerel

b. absorbed dose of x ray----gray

c. magnetic induction----weber

d. magnetic flux---tesla

e .frequency ---hertz

9.Following properties of EM radiation is explained by wave concept

a. reflection

b. refraction

c. diffraction

d. polarization

e. photoelectric effect

10.True regarding fundamental particles

a. neutron and proton has relative mass of 1

b. electron and positron has relative mass of 0.00054

c. alpha particle has relative mass of 2

d. proton and positron has relative charge of +1

e. alpha particle has relative charge of +4

11.True regarding Wilhelm Conrad Roentgen

a. Austrian physicist

b. discovered x ray on 8th Nov.1895

c. awarded the 1st Nobel Prize for physics

d. awarded the Nobel Prize in 1901

e. discovered x ray accidently

12. Members of family of Electromagnetic radiations are

a. x rays

b. radio waves

c.radiant heat

d. visible light

e. gamma radiation

13. True regarding EM radiation is/are

a. produced by accelerating charge outside atom

b. cyclotron is an accelerator that is EM radiation limited

c. produced in energy level transitions(including nuclear transitions

d. any accelerating charge not bound to an atom emit EM-radiation

e.x ray is an example of EM radiation

14.True regarding atom

a. nucleus positively charged due presence of positron

b. electrons orbits in specific shells

c. the shells are designated K,L,M,N—from periphery to centre

d. no valence shell can have more than eight electrons

e.the innermost shell is known as valence shell

15.True regarding basics of radiophysics

a. X-rays and gamma rays are an ionizing radiations

b. an atom consists mainly of filled space

c. protons and neutrons are together called nucleons

d. nuclide is a species of nucleus characterized by atomic number(p) and the mass number(p+n)

e. radionuclide is stable in nature

16.True regarding atom

a. innermost electron shell is

concerned with optical and electrical properties of the element

b. the properties of x ray and their interaction with materials concern with nucleus

c. radiactivity concerns orbiting electrons

d. outer electron shell is concerned with chemical and thermal properties of the element

e. metal 's good conduction of heat and electricity is due its free one,two or three electrons

17. True regarding atom/crystal

a. an atom is said to be ionized when one of electrons has been completely removed

b. ion pair refers to detached electron and remnant atom

c. silver bromide ,sodium iodide and cesium iodide are example of ionic crystal

d. electrostatic attraction holds the ionic component

e. silver bromide gas highly regular three-dimentional lattice

18. True regarding excited atom

a. raising of electron from from one shell to another further out

b. expenditure of energy in raising the electron

c. atom as a whole has less energy than normal

d. energy is remitted as a single packet of energy or photon of light(visible or ultraviolet)

e. example of quantum aspect of electromagnetic radiation

19. True matching regarding the binding energy(E_K kev) of different element

a. Aluminium   1.6
b. Molybdenum   20
c. Iodine   33
d. Barium   37
e. Gadolinium   50

20. Correct matching of SI unit

a. temperature ---- kelvin

b. energy ------joule ($1kg\ m^2\ s^{-2}$)

c. power-----watt ($1\ js^{-1}$)

d. electrical potential ---volt ($1j\ c^{-1}$)

e .luminous intensity ----candela

21. True regarding eV and units

a. eV energy acquired by an electron when accelerated through the potential difference of 1microvolt

b. $1\ e\ V = 1.6 \times 10^{-19}\ J$

c. SI unit of absorbed dose =gray

d. SI unit of radioactivity =Becquerel

e. SI unit of electric current = ampere

22. True regarding the binding energy of electron(E)

a. energy expanded in completely removing the electron

b. depend on shell ($E_K<E_L<E_M< ---$)

c. depend on the element ,increasing as the atomic number increases

d. E of tungsten ,$E_K= 70kev, E_L= 11kev$,$E_M=2kev$

e. E_k of lead $=88kev$

23. True regarding electromagnetic radiation

a. energy travelling across empty space

b. same velocity as light in vacuum

c. velocity very close to $3 \times 10^8 m/s$,but significantly less in air

d. x rays and gamma rays differ in their origin

e. x rays and gamma rays has different properties

24. correct matching of wavelength, frequency and

energy

a. radiowaves ---1000-0.1m,0.3-30000MHz,0.0001-10micro ev

b. visible light ---700-400nm,430-750THz,10-1000micro ev

c. ultraviolet –400-10nm,750-30000THz,1.8-100 ev

d. x rays and gamma rays—1-0.1pm ,3 x 10^5-3 x 10^9THz,1kev - 10Mev

e. infrared ---100-1micro,3-300THz,10-1000Mev

25.True regarding radiation

a. a collimated set of rays is called beam

b. photon fluence refers to number of photons /unit of cross sectional area at particular point

c. energy fluence refers to sum of energies of all individual photons/unit of cross sectional area

d. energy fluence rate/beam intensity refers to the total amount of energy /unit cross –sectional area/unit time

e. the intensity is proportional to the square of the amplitude

26.True regarding radiation

a. the photon energy is proportional to the frequency

b. photon energy (in kev)=1.24/frequency(in nm)

c .air kerma is inversely proportional to the square of the distance from the source.

 d. energy fluence and intensity are easy to measure directly

e. air kerma is an easier indirect measurement of energy fluence of X-rays and gamma rays

27. True regarding atoms is/are

a. J.J Thompson discovered electron in 1897

b .nucleons refers to elementary particles present in the nucleus

c. the neutrons and protons have same mass(1.66 x 10^{-24}gram)

d. mass of electron is 1836 times greater than than mass of an proton

e. the number of protons in the nucleus ia called the atomic number of the atom

28.True regarding wave aspects of electromagnetic radiation

a. longitudinal wave

b. the electric and magnetic vectors at right angle to each other

c. sinusoidal in nature

d. velocity of light in vaccum

e. wavelength x frequency =constant

29.True regarding electromagnetic spectrum

a. photon energy of radiowaves>microwaves>infrared>visible light>ultraviolet >x rays and gamma rays

b. frequency of radiowaves>microwaves>infrared>visible light>ultraviolet >x rays and gamma rays

c. wavelength of radiowaves>microwaves>infrared>visible light>ultraviolet >x rays and gamma rays

d. wavelength of radiowaves <microwaves<infrared<visible light<ultraviolet <x rays and gamma rays

e. photon energy of radiowaves<microwaves<infrared<visible light<ultraviolet <x rays and gamma rays

30.True regarding isotopes is/are

a. same number of protons

b. same atomic number
c. different numbers of neutrons
d. different atomic masses
e. different number of electrons

31.Number of electrons in different orbit.
a. 2 electrons in the first orbit (K)
b. upto 8 electrons in the second orbit (L)
c. upto 10 electrons in the third orbit (M)
d. upto 32 electrons in the fourth orbit (N)
e. upto 50 electrons in the second orbit (0)

32. Members of family of Electromagnetic radiations is/are
a. X- rays
b. radio waves
c. radiant heat
d. visible light
e. gamma radiation

33. True regarding EM radiation is/are
a. produced by accelerating charge outside atom
b. cyclotron is an accelerator that is EM radiation limited
c. produced in energy level transitions(including nuclear transitions
d. any accelerating charge not bound to an atom emit EM-radiation
e. x ray is an example of EM radiation

34. Correctly matched wavelengths of EM radiations is/are
a. soft x- rays==100 to 1 A^O
b. diagnostic x- rays==1 to 0.1 A^O
c. therapeutic x- rays==0.1 to 1^{-4} A^O
d. gamma rays==0.1 to 1^{-4} A^O
e. visible light ==75000 to 3900 A^O

Answer ---Basics Physics

1.abcde---- [Page 28/Christensen]

2.cde----The binding energy of K electrons shells varies from one element to another element .An electron of an atom can move from K shell to L shell by emission of energy .The diameter of the atom is about 100,000 times larger than the diameter of its its nucleus.The diameter of the nucleus of an atom is about 5×10^{-15m} and the diameter of the entire atom is about 5×10^{-10m}. [Page 28/Christensen]

3.abe-----Binding force the electron is inversely proportional to the square of the distance between the nucleus and electron,so K electron has larger binding force than an an L electron.Electrons in an atom is in negative energy states. [Page 27-28/Christensen]

4.abcd----Photons are discrete bundles of energy which depend on its frequency (E=Plank's constant x frequency,travels at the speed of light.The unit to measure the energy of photons is EV,ionizing radiation'photon energy is =>15 ev . [Page 6-7/Christensen]

5.abcd--- EM radiation can be propogated through a vaccum ,different EM radiations travels at the same velocity in a vacuum(3×10^8meters /sec ,186,000miles per second), differ basically in wavelengths only but there ia a considerable overlap in wavelengths of various members of EM spectrum . [Page 5 / Christensen]

6.bde----Regarding photon and ionizing radiation :Energy of photons in keV =24.2/wavelength(A^0),Plank's constant X frequency of photon give the energy of photons,an atom loses an electron on ionization, x ray energies are usually measured in EV,gamma rays and x rays and some ultraviolet rays are ionizing radiation. [Page 6-7/Christensen]

7.abcd--- EM radiation can be propogated through a vaccum ,different EM radiations travels at the same velocity in a vacuum(3×10^8meters /sec ,186,000miles per second), differ basically in wavelengths only but there ia a considerable overlap in wavelengths of various members of EM spectrum . [Page 5/Christensen]

8.abe----Correctly matched SI unit : radioactivity—Becquerel,absorbed dose of x ray----gray,magnetic induction----tesla,magnetic flux---weber,frequency ---hertz.[Page 8/Christensen]

9.abcd --- Properties of EM radiation explained by wave concept are reflection,refraction diffraction,polarization .The particle concept of EM radiation is used to describe the interactions between radiation and matter(photoelectric effect,Crompton'effect). [Page 6/Christensen]

10.abd---Alpha particle has relative charge of +2 and and relative mass of 4. (page 1/Farr)

11.bcde-- Wilhelm Conrad Roentgen: a German physicist,discovered X- ray on 8th Nov.1895 during investigation of behavior of cathode rays,was awarded the 1st Nobel Prize for physics in 1901 [Page 1/Christensen]

12.abcde----Members of family of Electromagnetic radiations are x rays,radio waves,radiant heat,visible light and gamma radiation. Elecromagnetic radiation is the transport of energy through space as a combination of electric and magnetic fields. [Page 1/Christensen]

13.abcde---- EM radiation is produced by accelerating charge outside atom ,also produced in energy level transitions(including nuclear transitions),any accelerating charge not bound to an atom(including the nucleus) emit EM-radiation.Cyclotron is an accelerator type that is EM radiation –limited. [Page 22/Christensen]

14.bd----Nucleus is positively charged due presence of proton.Electrons orbits in specific shells and the shells are designated K,L,M,N—ouward from centre .The outermost electrons are known as valence electrons. No valence shell can have more than eight electrons .Sodium atom has one electron in outermost shell,two electrons in K-shell ,eight in the L-shell (page no.2/Farr)

15.acd-----An atom consists mainly of empty space.Radionuclide is unstable in nature and so radioactive . (page no.1/Farr)

16.de---The properties of x ray and their interaction with materials concern with orbiting electrons particularly those in inner shell.Radiactivity concerns with nucleus. (page no.2/Farr)

17.abcde---- (Chapter 1,page no.3,second edition (2008),Farr's Physics for Medical Imaging)

18.bde---excitation of atom involves raising of electron from one shell to another further out with expenditure of energy so atom as a whole has more energy than normal.(page no.3/Farr)

19.abcde ----(page no.3/Farr)

20.abcde------(page no.2/Farr)

21.bcde---e V refers to energy acquired by an electron when accelerated through the potential difference of 1 volt. (page no.2/Farr)

22.acde---- The binding energy of electron(E) depend on shell $(E_K>E_L>E_M> --)$(page no.3/Farr)

23.abd---- Electromagnetic radiation is a term given to energy travelling across empty space has same velocity as light in vacuum ,velcity very close to 3×10^8m/s and not significantly less in air.X- rays and gamma rays have essentially the same properties . (page no.3/Farr)

24.abcde------(page no.4/Farr)

25.abcde---(page no.4/Farr)

26.abce--- Energy fluence and intensity are not easy to measure directly. ---(page no.4-5/Farr)

27.abce----Mass of proton is 1836

times greater than mass of an proton. (page no.27/Farr)

28.bcde----Electromagnetic radiation is a longitudinal wave . (page no.4/Farr)

29.abd---(page no.4/Farr)

30.abcd---Isotopes of an element has same number of electrons. [Page 27/Christensen]

31.abde---Number of electrons ,upto 10 electrons in the third orbit (M) . [Page 27/Christensen]

32. abcde----Members of family of Electromagnetic radiations are x-rays, radio waves, radiant heat, visible light and gamma radiation. Elecromagnetic radiation is the transport of energy through space as a combination of electric and magnetic fields.

[Page 1/Christensen]

33.abcde---- EM radiation is produced by accelerating charge outside atom , produced in energy level transitions(including nuclear transitions). Any accelerating charge not bound to an atom (including the nucleus) emit EM-radiation. Cyclotron is an accelerator type that is EM radiation –limited. [Page 2/Christensen]

34.abcde--- Wavelengths of EM radiations :soft x rays==100 to 1 A^O,diagnostic x rays==1 to 0.1 A^O,therapeutic x rays==0.1 to 1^{-4} A^O,gamma rays==0.1 to 1^{-4} A^O,visible light ==75000 to 3900 A^O [Page 6/Christensen]

CHAPTER 2

X- Ray tube and X-Ray production

1.True regarding X-ray tube
a.tube eneryy is supplied by DC mains by means of transformer
b.tube current is contolled by adjusting the filament voltage and filament current
c.A small increase in filament temperature produce no effect over tube current
d.increasing or decreasing the tube voltage does not affect the tube current
e.tube voltage is unaffected by changes in the tube filament

2.True regarding the x-ray generator
a.produce high voltage to be applied between the anode and cathode
b.single –phase ,self –rectified generator produce tube current during the negative phase of the kilovoltage cycle
c. single –phase ,self –rectified generator,is commonly used generator in ophthalmic radiography
d.the time between peaks is 20ms for the 50 Hz mains frequency used in the UK
e.Rectification convert AC into pulsating direct current

3.True regarding tube current ia/are
a.refers to the number of electrons flowing /sec from the filament to the target
b.The number(quantity) of x rays produced depends entirely on the tube current

c.electrons are produced at the filament by thermionic emission
d.the connecting wires supply both the voltage (average 10v) and the amperage(average about 3-5A)
e.Edison effect refers to the electron cloud surrounding the filament

4.True regarding radiography
a.macroradiography helpful for visualizing small detail
b.macroradiography is generally used only in mammography
c.distortion refers to a difference between the shape of a structure in the image and in the object
d.distortion may be due to foreshortening ofr differential magnification
e.distortion is reduced by using shorter FFD

5.True regarding x ray tube is/are of [Chapter 2,Page 11, Christensen's Physics of Diagnostic radiology]
a.the tungsten filament must be at least heated to 2200^{0C} for emission useful no.of electrons
b.space charge refers to electrons cloud in the immediate vicinity of filament
c.electron current across an x ray tube is in either direction
d.tube current of 100 milliamperes means flow of $6.25x\,10^{17}$ electrons per 1 sec

e.Tungsten is more efficient than its allow for emitting electrons

6.True regarding focal spot

a.actual focal spot is area over which heat is produced

b.actual focal spot determines the tube rating

c.the target angle is generally between 7-10 degree

d.the smaller the target angle ,the greater is the forshortening of foacl spot

e.use of a steeper target serves to decrease the target heat rating for a given effective focal spot.

7.True regarding intensifying screen

a.x ray film is used with a pair of screen

b.front screen absorbs a half of the xray radition falling on the front screen

c.half of the light produced by the front screen exposes the front emulsion

d.the rear screen absorbs about a half of the X-ray radiation transmitted by the front screen

e.intensifying screen uses phosphorescence material to erase the memory

8.Regarding x ray tube

a.may have two or three filament

b.two focal spots used in stereoscopic angiographic tube

c.automatic filament-boosting circuit is used to prolong tube's life

d.aging tubes becomes bronze-colored

e.vaporization alter the quality of x ray and increase possibility of arcing

9.Regarding X ray tube and production

a.most of energy of electrons is converted into heat

b.>10% of energy of electorns is converted into x rays

c.it is best to keep the temperature of tungsten anode below 2000^0c

d.line focus principle cause apparent increase in focal spot size

e.the melting point of tungsten is about 3370^0c

10.True regarding stationary anode of x ray tube

a.made of tungsten

b.2-3 mm thick plate

c.rectangular or square

d.each dimension of plate >1cm

e.embedded in a large mass of cupper

11.Reasons for chosing Tungsten as the target material is/are.

a.high atomic number (74) ,so more efficient for the production of x rays

b.high melting points (3370^0c),so withstand the high temperature produced

c.reasonably good material for the absorption of heat

d.reasonably good material for the rapid dissipation of the heat away from the target area

d.cheap and widely available

12.True regarding effect of the tube current(m A) and atomic number of the target

a.increasing the tube current alter the shape of the spectrum

b.increasing the tube current increase the output of bremstrahlung only

c.lowering the atomic number of target reduce output of bremsstrahlung

d. lowering the atomic number of target alter shape of bremsstrahlung if filtration is changed.

e. lowering the atomic number of target reduce the photon energy of the characteristic lines .

13.True regarding the tube potential waveform (kv waveform)

a. tube potential waveform (kv waveform) produce no change in the maximum and minimum photon energies

b.more x rays are produced by a constant or three phase generator

c.more output are by produced a constant or three phase generator

d. higher energies x ray are produced by a constant or three phase generator

e. x rays of greater the effective energy are by produced a constant or three phase generator

14.True regarding anode in x ray tube is/are

a.Tungsten target is embedded in a large mass of copper

b.copper increase the thermal capacity of the anode and speed its rate of cooling

c.melting point of copper is 2300^0c

d.the actual size of target is considerably smaller than the area of electron bombardment

e.copper and tungsten has different coefficients of expansion

15.True regarding rotating anode

a.make tube capable of withastanding high generated heat

b.theoretically rotate at 3000 rpm

c.beveled edge in tungsten disc

d.spread the heat produced during an exposure

e.the diameter of the tungsten disc affects the maximum permissible loading of the anode

16.True regarding rotating anode

a.stator coils and the induction motor provide the power to rotate the anode assembly

b.Grahite is used as lubricant in bearings

c.heat dissipisation is by absorption and conduction

d.the stem is made of molybdenum for its high metlting point and poor heat conduction

e.the stem is made as short as possible

17.True regarding rotating anode

a.in Tungsten-rhenium anode ,roughening and pitting is a major problem

b.molybdenum and graphite are used in tungsten anode to reduce its inertia

c.slits or grooves in the target surface is of no benefit

d.blackening of back of the anode aids in heat dissipation

e.specific gravity of molybdenum is more than tungsten

18.True regarding Grid-controlled X-ray tube

a.allow the x ray tube to be turned on and off rapidly

b.used in cinefluorography

c.the focusing cup is used as a third electrode

d.focusing cup is electrically positive relative to the filament

e.the voltage applied between the focusing cup and the anode act like a switch

19.True regarding space charge in X-ray tube

a.residual space charge exist around filament above the saturation voltage

b.the tube current increase as tube voltage is increased upto saturation voltage

c.the tube current is emission – limited /temperature limited below the saturation voltage

d.the space charge effect has, theoretically ,no influence on the tube current above the saturation voltage

e.Different X-ray tube has different saturation voltages and require different amounts of space charge compensation

20.True regarding Heel effect

a.Heel effect refers to variation in intensity of the x ray beam that leaves the x ray tube

b.due to angling of cathode

c.more intensity of x ray beam toward the cathode side of tube

d.more noticeable when larger focus-film distance used

e.Heel effect less for smaller film for equal target-film distance

21.True regarding the X- ray tube housing

a.lined with lead

b.absorb primary and secondary x rays

c.provide shielding for the high voltages

d. extremely thick mineral oil between the x ray tube the housing

e.the oil provide continuous lubrication for the rotating node

22.The parameter that measures x-ray tube loading is/are

a.the heat unit

b.the watt-second/joule

c.kilowatt rating

d.rem

e.sievert

23.True regarding attenuation is/are

a.the unit of the coefficient is the reciprocal of the unit of the absorber

b.the mass attenuation coefficient is same for water ,ice and vapour

c. mass attenuation coefficient is independent of the density of the absorber

d.increasing the radiation energy decreases attenuation

e.increasing the density decreases attenuation

24.True regarding x ray tube is/are.

a.maximum temperature to which tungsten can be safely raised is 2000^0c

b.considerable vaporization of tungsten occurs above 3000^0c

c.the total heat produced in x ray tube is a product of votage,current and exposure time

d.the peak voltage in single -phase generator is 1.4 or 1.35 times the average voltage

e.Heat unit is defined for triple phase generator

25.In the equation $N=N_0e^{-mu \times k}$, symbols used are

a.N stands for the number of incident photons

b.N_O stands foe the number of transmitted photons

c.e stands for base of natural logarithm

d.mu. stands for linear attenuation coefficient

e.k stands for absorber thickness in

cm

26. True regarding metal/ceramic X- ray tubes

a. metal incasing
b. two ceramic insulators
c. cathode rotate on an axle
d. ceramic insulators insulate the high voltage parts of the x ray tube
e. permit use of massive anode ,to the extent of 2kg

27. True regarding Compton effect

a. due to interaction of x ray photon with a loosely bound or free electron
b. bounces off a free electron
c. recoil electron energy depend on the angle of scattering
d. electrons may be scattered in all directions
e. the photons are projected only in sideways and forwards directions

28. Advantages of metal incasing is/are

a. less off- focus radiation
b. longer tube life
c. high tube currents
d. higher tube loading
e. adequate electrical safety

29. True regarding off focus radiation is/are

a. due to interaction of high speed electrons with metal surfaces other than the focal track of the anode
b. the main source of off-focus electrons is electron backscatter from the anode
c. off-focus radiation may be partly controlled by palcing the collimator or a lead diaphragm
d. the metal enclosure decreases off-focus radiation
e. there is more off-focus radiation

in metal x ray tube than glass one

30. True regarding process of X-ray generation.

a. fast moving electrons interact with the tungsten target
b. One electron volt =1.6 x 10^{-19} J
c. 100 kVp means the minimum voltage across the tube is 100,000 V
d. the voltage providing the potential to accelerate the electrons is pulsating
e. the high speed electrons striking the target donot have the same energy

31. True regarding general radiation (bremsstrahlung)

a. involves interaction of speeding electrons with nucleus of target tungsten
b. there is a wide distribution in the energy of general radiation
c. the maximum wavelength(lowest energy) in general radiation depend on the x ray tube voltage(kVp)
d. 99% of all reactions in general radiation produce heat
e. bremsstrahlung is a German term means 'braking radiation'

32. True regarding x ray production

a. the ejection of Auger electrons produce characteristic radiation
b. the energy lost during interaction of electron with the nucleus produce characteristic radiation
c. the alpha$_1$ and alpha$_2$ characteristic x rays arise from transition of M – shell electrons to the K-shell
d. the beta$_1$ characteristic x rays arise from transition of L–shell electrons to the K-shell
e. the beta$_2$ characteristic x rays arise from transition of an N –shell

electrons to the K-shell

33.Factors affecting the intensity of the x ray beam as/are

a.the kilovoltage

b.x ray tube current

c.the target material

d.the filtration

e.cathode filament

34.Regarding intensity of X-ray beam

a.for continuous spectrum ,the atomic number of the target material partly determines the quantity of a x-ray produced

b.the atomic number of the target material determines the energy or quality of characteristic x rays produced

c.With tungsten anode ,the x ray beam consists almost entirely of characteristic radiation

d.The kVp determines the minimum energy (quality) of the x rays produced

e.the amount of radiation produced increases as the square of the kilovoltage

35.Tungsten is chosen for use in x ray tube because of

a.can be drawn into thin wire

b.can be drawn into strong wire

c.has a high melting point(2370^{0C})

d.has little tendency to vaporize

e.has relatively long life expectancy

36.Correct matching of atomic number and melting point

Atomic numbe / melting point

a.tungsten   74 /3370^{0}c

b.platinum   78 /1770^{0}c

c.gold   79/1063^{0}c

d.tungsten   74 /2370^{0}c

e.platinum   78 /3370^{0}c

37.True regarding x ray photons

interaction with matter

a.interact with orbital electrons or nucleus

b.interactions are always with nucleus, in the diagnostic energy range

c.photoelectric effect , Compton scattering ,pair production are pattern of interaction

d.scatter radiation improves contrast

e.in coherent scattering ,radiation undergoes a change in direction without a change in wavelength.

38.True regarding coherent scattering/unmodified scattering /classical scattering

a.change in direction without change in wavelength

b.single electron of atom involved in Thomson scattering

c.all electrons of an atom involved in Rayleigh scattering

d. involve energy transfer and ionization

e.produce film fog,so important in diagnostic radiology

39.True regarding atoms

a.the innermost shell is called the K shell

b.each shell has limited electron capacity

c.each shell has a specific binding energy

d.electrons in the outermost cell are tightly bound

e.atomic number does not influence the binding energy of shell

40.True regarding characteristic curve

a.show response of a film and screen combination to X-rays

b.graph of optical density as a function of exposure plotted on a linear scale

c.densitometer is used to derive characteristic curve

d.the toe is high-density region in which the slope of curve is shallow

e.the shoulder is the region of correct exposure

41.True regarding photoelectric effect

a.the incident photon energy should be more than the binding energy of electrons

b. produce a photoelectron that has great penetrating capacity

c.the incident photon is deflected in photoelectric effect

d.characteristic radiation is produced

e.produce a positive ion

42.True regarding induction motor

a.induction motor rotate the anode with relatively friction free mechanical linkage

b.induction motor contain stator coils in which AC current flow

c.there is no time delay before anode comes up to its full speed

d.High speed anodes are energized with three-phase mains and rotate at 9000rpm.

e.anode stops immediately after static coils are de-enerzised

43.True regarding photoelectric effect

a.more likely to occur when the photon energy and electron binding energy are nearly same with photon energy greater than the binding energy

b.photoelectric effect is inversely proportional to approx.the third power of energy

c.the tighter an electron is bound in its orbit ,the more likely it is to be involved in a photoelectric reaction

d.the photoelectric effect is roughly proportional to the third power of the atomic number

e.the photoelectric effect cannot occur with a free electron

44. correct matching

Atomic number/k-shell binding energy(keV)

a.aluminium   13/1.56
b.iodine   53/33.2
c.barium   56/37.4
d.tungsten   74/69.5
e.lead   82/88.0

45.True regarding photoelectric reactions

a.the photoelectric effect produces scatter radiation

b.enhances natural tissue contrast

c.produrce radiographic images of excellent quality

d.patient receives more radiation than from any other type of interaction

e. most common with low energy photons and high atomic number absorbers

46.True regarding Compton scattering

a.responsible for almost all the scatter radiation in diagnostic radiology

b.interaction of relatively low energy incident photons with outer shell electron

c.the incident photon loses all the energy in the process

d.the recoil electron appear as scatter radiation

e.an ion pair is produced

47.True regarding Compton

effect

a.no energy is expanded in freeing electron

b.with x ray energies of 1MeV, most scattered photons deflect in a forward direction

c.in diagnostic energy range ,the scattered photons has relatively symmetrical distribution

d.upto 150keV ,the incident photons retains most of original energy

e.at wide angle of deflection ,scattered photons retain almost all their original energy

48.True regarding scattered radiation with narrow angle of deflection

a.retain almost all their original energy

b.no chance of reaching x-ray film and producing fog

c.removed by filters

d.removed by grids

e.not a problem in diagnostic radiology

49.Requirements of material for anode is /are

a.a high conversion efficiency for electrons into x rays

b.high atomic number

c.high melting point

d.high conductivity

e.a low vapor pressure

50.True regarding Compton reaction

a.probability of Compton reaction depend on the total number of electrons

b.the number of Compton reaction is dependent on the atomic number of the absorber

c.the number of Compton reaction

gradually increase as photon energy increases

d.probability of Compton reaction depend on density of the absorber

e.Compton effect is not a issue in fluoroscopy

51.True regarding heel effect

a.less intensity of x rays towards the cathode edge

b.steeper the target, the greater is the heel effect

c.reduced heel effect for a given film size at longer FFD

d.roughening increases the heel effect

e.place the thicker part of patients towards cathode side

52.True regarding anode cooling

a.heat produced on the focal track is conducted quickly into the anode disk

b.Heat from anode disk is transferred by radiation to the insulating oil

c.rotor is always in danger of overheating and seizing up

d.blackening the anode assembly promote the radiation

e.the rate of heat radiation decreases as the anode assembly gets hotter

53.True regarding radiation interaction

a.pair production does not occur with photon energies less than 1.02 MeV

b.photodisintegration doesnot occur with energies less than 7MeV

c.part of nucleus in form of neutron/proton/alpha particle is ejected by high energy photon

d.the photon interact with nucleus in pair production

e.positron and electron are

produced in pair production

54. True regarding X-ray tube

a.the filament voltage is about 10 V

b.the filament current is about 10 A

c.the accelerating voltage/tube potential/high voltage/kilovoltage/kv 30 to 150 kv

d.typical tube current /milliamperage/m A 0.5-1000 m A

e.typical temperature of cathode 2200 degree Celsius

55. True regarding x- ray tubes is/are

a.diode tube containing two electrodes

b.made of pyrex glass

c.filled with neutral gas argon

d.electrons produced at anode

e.x-rays produced at cathode.

56. True regarding intensity of x ray

a.the wavelength of characteristic x ray depend upon the kVp

b.greater the m A ,more is x rays produced

c.the quality of x ray depend almost entirely on the x ray tube current

d.heat production in the x ray tube is minimized by using the line focus principle and a rotating anode

e.molybdunum anode producing charecteristic radiation (17.5 and 19.6 keV) makes up significant portion of the total radiation

57. True regarding x-ray tube is/are

a.vaccum in x-ray tube allow the number and the speed of the accelerating electrons to be controlled independently.

b.The negative terminal of the x ray tube is called the anode

c.the cathode consists of filament ,connecting wires and focusing cup

d.the filament is made of tungsten wire

e.the connecting wire and pyrex glass has different coefficients of linear expansion.

58. True regarding generator

a.6 pulses and 12 pulses three-phase generator has associated ripple theoretically equal to 13% and 4% respectively

b.high –frequency generator has ripple factor of no more than 1%

c.modern X-ray equipment uses high –frequency generators

d.high frequency generators first convert mains AC into high frequency AC (M>/=1kHz)

e.high frequency generators are particularly compact and stable

59. True regarding X ray tube processes

a.electrons strikes the target with kinetic energy equivalent to half of the tube potential

b.the electrons penetrate several millimeters into the target

c.the electrons produce heat on interacting with inner electrons of the atom

d.electrons produce X rays by interating with inner shells of atom

e. electrons produce X rays by interacting with of the field of nucleus

60. True regarding film processing

a.use alkaline solution of thiosulphate ('hypo')

b.fixer dissolves out the unaffected silver ions

c.the image is stable and unaffected by light after fixation

d.washing is done to remove retained hypo

e.vinegary smell in the stored film may be due to retained silver ion

61.True regarding optical density

a. developed x ray film is negative image

b.optical density /blackening of an area of the film depends on the number of silver grains per unit area

c.optical density is defined as the log of the ratio of the intensities of the incident and transmitted light

d.optical density is measured by dosimeter

e.the density of the area of interest on a properly exposed film averages about 3

62.True regarding characteristic radiation

a.energy of K_{alpha} and K_{beta} radiation of tungsten are 58kev and 68kev respectively

b. energy of K_{alpha} and K_{beta} radiation of molybdenum are 17.5 kev and 20 kev respectively

c.the photon energy of the K radiation decrease as the atomic number of target increases

d.characteristic radiation is produced when tube voltage and so maximum energy of electrons exceed the E_k

e.the rate of production of characteristic radiation decreases as the kv increases above E_k

63.True regarding x ray tube and its process

a.x rays and gamma rays are ionizing radiation

b.E_k of tungsten is 88 kev

c. anode emit electons

d.characteristic radiation energy is determined by the target material

e.80 % or more of x ray emitted by diagnostic x ray tube are characterisc in nature

64.True regarding bremsstrahlung(breaking radiation)

a.X rays produced by interaction of electron with the nucleus

b.In mammography ,bremssstrahlung is responsible for 80% of the emitted xrays

c.the bremsstrahlung forms a continuous spectrum

d.the maximum photon energy (in kev) is numerically equal to the half of tube potential (kv)

e.there is no low- energy cut off .

65.True regarding the X-ray spectrum

a.the peak of continuous spectrum (the most common photon energy) is typically between one-third and one-half of the tube potential

b.the average /effective energy of photon is between 50-60% of the maximum

c.the area of the spectrum represents the total output of all X – rays photons emitted

d.increase in tube voltage increases both the width and height of the spectrum

e.the intensity of the emitted x rays is approximately proportional to (tub voltage)^2 x m A (in tube range of 60- 120 kv)

66.Regarding performance tests on the x ray tube and generator

a. a metal frame generally 150mm square is used to test light baem diaphragm alignment and bucky centering

b.the kv is generally measured indirectly using a pentrameter

c.the output of the tube can be measured using a dosimeter,often an ionization chamber

d.step wedge made of aluminium may be used to as simple alternative to the use of kv meter and ionization chamber

e.focal spot size measured using a pinhole camera or a star test tool.

67.True regarding effects of tube potential(kv)

a.increasing the kv shifts the x ray spectrum and upwards and to the right

b.increasing the kv increases the maximum energy of x ray photons

c.increasing the kv decreases the effective energies of x ray photons

d.increasing the kv increases the total number of x ray photons

e.increasing the kv decreases the efficiency of x ray production.

68.True regarding interaction of x ray and gamma rays with matte

a.scattering and absorption are only two possible fate in interaction with matter

b.x-ray absorption and scattering processes are stochastic processes

c.The x ray images is formed by the absorbed photons

d.photons absorbed and scattered represent attenuation by the matter

e.HVL is a measure of the penetrating power or effective energy of the beam

69.True regarding the half –value layer (HVL)

a.refers to density of the stated material

b.reduce the the intensity of x ray beam to one half of its originals

c.measure of the penetrating power or effective energy of the beam

d.HVL=0.693 linear attenuation coefficient

e.HVL can be used for monoenergetic beams only

70.True regarding linear attenuation coefficient

a.measure the probability of interaction of photon with specified material

b.applies only to narrow monoenergetic beam

c.coefficient increases as the density and the atomic number increases

d.coefficient increases as photon energy increases

e.the mass attenuation coefficient is independent of density of material

71.True regarding attenuation

a.the x ray can be completely absorbed in a material

b.graph of percentage transmission versus thickness of material   is an exponential curve

c.logarathmic scale graph of percentage transmission versus thickness of material is a straight line

d. a norrow beam is used for the measurement of the half value layer

e.measured HVL would be smaller in case of use of wide beam

72.True regarding attenuation

a.the HVL of a typical diagnostic beam is 30mm in tissue ,12mm in bone and 0.15 mm in lead

b.increase in the proportion of higher energy photons during its passage though the matter is known as beam hardening beam

c.interaction with a loosely bound or free electron is usually reffered as the Compton effect (inelastic/non-coherent scattering)

d.interaction with an inner shell or bound electron is known as photoelectric absorption

e.interaction with a bound electron is known as elastic scatter

73.True regarding Compton effect

a.greater the angle of scattering,the lesser the energy and range of the recoil of electron

b. greater the angle of scattering,the greater the loss of energy of the scattered photon

c. greater the angle of scattering,the greater wavelength of the scattered photon

d.the higher the initial initial photon energy ,the lesser the remaining photon energy of the scattered radiation

e. the higher the initial initial photon energy ,the more penetrating the scattered energy

74.True regarding scattered electons

a.energy of back -scattered electron < side electron <forward electron

b.energy of back -scattered electron < side electron> forward electron

c.enrgy of back -scattered electron > side electron> forward electron

d.energy of back -scattered electron = side electron> forward electron

e.energy of back -scattered electron > side electron =forward electron

75.True regarding the Compton process

a.proportional to the physical density (mass/unit volume)

b.proportional to electron density

c.independent of the atomic number of material

d.decreases only slightly over the range of photon energies of diagnostic radiology

e.very approximately proportional to $1/E$(binding energy)

76.True regarding Compton process

a.the softening effect of Compton scatter is greatest with small scattering angles as well as with high energies X-rays

b.the electron density of bone ,air ,fat ,muscle and water does not vary more than 1%

c.the mass attenuation coefficient for the Compton effect is the same within 30% for air ,tissue ,bone,contrast media and lead

d.the energy carried off by the recoil electron is said to have been absorbed by the material

e.in diagnostic range ,no more than 20% of the energy is absorbed ,the rest being scattered

77.True regarding photoelectric effect

a.photon x- ray with energy more than E_K eject an electron from the k-shell

b.the energy of the photon is incompletely absorbed in the process

c.the kinetic energy of photoelectron= photon energy – E_k/E_L

d.characteristic radiation has very low energy in low atomic number material as tissue

28

e.low energy characteristic radiation is absorbed completely with ejection of a further ,low energy or Auger electron

78.True regarding intensifying screen

a.the intensity of light emotted by a screen depends on the phosphor

b.the color of light emitted by the phosphor depends on activator

c.the spectral sensitivity of the film should not match the spectral emission of the screen

d.calcium tungstate emits a continouous spectrum of violet and red light

e.ordinary x ray film is sensitive to ultraviolet and blue light

79.True regarding photoelectric process.

a.inversely proportional to the cube of the photon energy E

b.proportional to the cube of the atomic number

c.proportional to the density of the material

d.the effective atomic number is defined as the cube root of the weighted sum of the cube of the atomic numbers of the constituents

e.the Compton and photoelectric interactions depend on the effective atomic number but not on the molecular configuration

80.True regarding effective atomic number

a.a mixture or compound has an effective atomic number

b.refers to average of the atomic numbers of the constituent elements

c.effective atomic number of fat,air and atomic number is 6.4,7.6 and

7.4 respectively

d.effective atomic number of bone is 13.3

e.the Compton ,not photoelectric interaction depend on the effective atomic number

81.True regarding cassette

a.light-permissible box

b.the front cassette is made of low atomic material ,possibly carbon fibre

c.the cassette back usually incorporates a thin lead sheet

d.the front screen nature is particularly important in mammograpgy

e.the cassette back material nature is meant to minimize backscattered radiation

82.True regarding absorption edges

a.when the photon energy reaches E_k, the probability of photoelectric absorption slumps to a lower level (K-absorption edge)

b.the probability of photoelectric absorption increases as photon energy increases further beyond the E_k

c.the K-absorption edge occurs at different photon energies with different materials

d.the higher the atomic number ,the lower is the photon energy at which the edge occurs

e.E_k of iodine =33kev

83.True regarding focusing cup is/are

a.surrounds the anode

b.usually made of nickel

c. has positive potential

d.converge electrons onto the anode

e.prevent spread of electons

84. True regarding absorption edge

a. the K-edge of low atomic atomic number materials(air ,water,tissue ,aluminium) have no significance

b. important for choosing materials for the X-ray beam filter

c. important for choosing materials for contrast media

d. important for choosing material for imaging phosphor

e. a material is relatively opaque to ints own characteristic radiation

85. True regarding interaction

a. the photoelectric coefficient is proportional to Z^3/E^3

b. the photoelectric coefficient is high when photon energy is just lesser than E_k

c. the Compton coefficient is independent of Z(atomic number) but largely affected by E

d. the photoelectric absorption is more important than the Compton process with high Z materials and with high energy photons

e. the photon energy at which the photoelectric and Compton process are equally important are about 30 kev for air ,water and tissue, 50 kev for aluminium and bone

86. True regarding interaction

a. the Compton process is the predominant process for air ,water and soft tissue

b. photoelectric absorption predominates for contrast material ,lead

c. photoelectric absorption predominates in materials used in films and screen

d. the Compton process and photoelectric absorption,both are important for bone

e. elastic scattering occurs if the photon energy is less than the binding energy of the electron

87. True regarding secondary electrons

a. refers to recoil elecrons and photoelectrons set moving in the material by Compton and photoleclectric process

b. interact with inner shells of nearby atom and cause excitation and ionization

c. the greater the initial energy of the electron ,the greater is its range

d. the range is directly proportional to the density of the material

e. the track of electron is dotted with ion pairs

88. True regarding secondary electrons

a. when travelling through air,the electron loses an average of 34 ev per ion pair formed

b. 3 ev is needed to excite an atom in air

c. about 10ev needed to ionize an atom in air

d. about eight times exitations as ionizations

e. th range in air is some 800 times greater than in tissue

89. Excitations and ionizations by the secondary electrons serves basis of

a. the measurement of x rays and gamma rays

b. biological damage

c. luminescence ,scintillation,fluorescence

d. basis of conventional radiography

e. heating in the material

90. True regarding ionising

radiations

a.x rays and gamma rays are indirectly ionizing agents

b.alpha is directly ionizing agents

c.some of ultraviolet radiations are ioninsing in nature

d. neutrons are indirectly ionizing agents

e. beta particle are directly ionizing agents

91.True regarding attenuation in radiology

a.the intensity of a beam is product of the number(quantity) and energy(quality) of the photons

b.refers to reduction in the intensity of an x ray beam as it traverses through the the the x ray tube and plate.

c.due to absorption or deflection in the x ray beam as it traverses through the matter

d.depends on both the quantity and the quality of the radiation

e.quality doesnot change on attenuation in case of monochromatic radiation

92.True regarding rare earth phosphor screen

a.are elements with atomic numbers (57-70) and K-edges (31-61keV)

b.less efficient than calcium tungstate

c.less sensitive(faster) than calcium tungstate screen

d.require smaller dose that is 2-3 times lower than calcium tungstate

e.phosphors incorporate no impurities

93.True regarding attenuation of monochromatic radiation

a.reduction in quantity (no of photons)

b.reduction of quality (energies)

c. arithmetic attenuation as passes through the matter

d. straight line on semi-logarithmic graph

e.the attenuation coefficient measure of attenuation

94.Regarding attenuation constant

a.the division of the linear attenuation coefficient by half-value layer is equal to 0.693

b.the half value layer is the absorber thickness required to reduce the intensity of the original beam by one half

c.half value layer is a common method for expressing the quality of an x ray beam

d.beam with high half value layer is less penetrating than one with a low half value layer

e.mass attenuation coefficient is obtained by dividing the linear attenuation coefficient by the density (cm^2/cm)

95.In the equation $N=N_0 e^{-mu \times k}$, symbols used are

a.N stands for the number of incident photons

b.N_O stands foe the number of transmitted photons

c.e stands for base of natural logarithm

d.mu. stands for linear attenuation coefficient

e.k stands for absorber thickness in cm

96.True regarding attenuation is/are

a.the unit of the coefficient is the reciprocal of the unit of the absorber

b.the mass attenuation coefficient is

same for water ,ice and vapour

c. mass attenuation coefficient is independent of the density of the absorber

d.increasing the radiation energy decreases attenuation

e.increasing the density decreases attenuation

97.True regarding relationship of energy of beam ,atomic number and type of interaction

a.with increase in radiation energy ,the percentage of photoelectric reaction decreases for water and bone

b.with increase in atomic number,the percentage of photoelectric reactions increase

c.with extremely low energy radiation as 20 keV ,the photoelectric reaction predominates regardless of the atomic number of the absorber

d.with sodium iodide ,photoelectric effect is the predominant interaction throughout the diagnostic energy range

e.attenuation is always greater when the photoelectric effect predominates

98.True regarding atomic number and interaction

a.with high atomic number absorber,transmission of radiation beam may paradoxically decrease with increasing energy

b.a sudden reduction in radiation transmission through lead occurs at 88keV due to Compton effect

c.gram for gram,lead is better absorber of x rays then the tin between 29-88 keV.

d.Iodine and barium has ideal K-

shell binding energies for interaction with diagnostic range x beam

e.when maximum x ray absorption is desired,the K-edge of an absorber should be closely matched with to the energy of the x ray beam.

99.Correct matching of atomic number and K-edge(keV)

a.Beryllium   4/11

b.aluminium   13/1.6

c.copper   29/9

d.zinc   30/9.7

e.selenium   32/11.1

100.Correct matching of atomic number and K-edge(keV)

a.molybdenum 42/20

b.tin   50/29.1

c.iodine   53/33.2

d.baruim   56/37.4

e.lead   82/88

101.True regarding density and interaction

a.density determines the tissue's stopping power

b.determines the number of electrons present in a given thickness

c.there is non linear relationship between density and attenuation

d.the number of Compton reaction depend on the number of electrons present in a given thickness

e.absorbers with many electrons are less impervious to radiation than absorbers with few electrons

102.True regarding electrons /gram and interaction

a.the bone has more electron/gram than water

b.the relative number of electrons per gram is calculated by number of electrons/weight of the atom

c.lead has more electrons per gram

than oxygen

d.In general ,the high atomic number elements has about 20% more electrons than the low atomic number elements

e.The effective atomic number of water and bone is 7.42 and 13.8 respectively

103.True regarding polychromatic radiation is/are.

a.the energy of the most energetic photon is determined by mAs

b.the mean energy is between one third and one half of its peak energy

c.mean energy of photons decreases as a result of attenuation

d.undergo change in quantity as well as quality during attenuation

e.high energy photons are initially eliminated during attenuation

104.True statements are

a.the film appears white when all the photons are transmitted

b.contrast is reduced if the differential attenuation is less

c.the differential attenuation depends entirely upon density when the Compton reactions is predominant.

d.with increase of photon energy (20 to100 keV) ,the Compton linear attenuation for bone decreases by 20%

e.fat and water can be differentiated by photoelectric attenuation using low energy techniques

105.True regarding scatter radiation

a.contributes no useful information

b.source is Compton scattering

c.the most important factor in its production is field size

d.there is a plateau to its production

as field size ,part thickness is increased

e.the quantity of scatter radiation continues to increase with increasing beam energy

106.True regarding line focus principle in x ray tube is/are

a.line focus principle cause apparent decrease in focal spot size

b.anode angle refers to angle the anode forms with the plane perpendicular to the incident electron beam

c.as the anode angle is made smaller ,the apparent focal size becomes larger

d.there is limit to decrease to anode angle due to the Heel effect(the point of anode cutoff)

e.0.3mm focal spot refers to its actual size

107.True regarding geometrical unsharpness

a.geometrical unsharpness =focal spot x object film distance /film-focus distance —object film distance

b.reduced by a smaller focal spot

c.reduced by decreasing the object-film distance

d.reduced by a longer FFD

e.related to the image of moving structures

108.The factors controlling the X ray spectrum.

a.the tube potential

b.the tube current

c.atomic number of the target

d.the tube potential waveform

e.filtration

109.True regarding focal spot

a.the steeper the target ,the narrower the useful x rays and the smaller the field covered b.a steep target is appropriate in mammography and in cardiac angiography

c.larger focal spot is used for improved resolution

d.focal spot size is constant

e.typical focal spot size for mammography is 0.6-1.2 mm

110. True regarding focal spot

a.it is not constant in size

b.depend upon m A and kv

c.blooming refers to less effective focusing of electron beam as m A increases

d.blooming becomes more significant at lower settings of KV

e.steep target is appropriate in mammography

111. True regarding rotating anode

a.bevelled disc

b.anode disk ,7-10cm in diameter

c.anode disk usually made of molybdenum/graphite

d.the target usually an allow of tungsten and rhenium

e.silver used as lubrication

112. True rotating anode

a.alloy of tungsten and rhenium has better thermal characteristics than pure tungsten

b.alloy of tungsten and rhenium doesnot roughen with use as quickly as tungsten

c.stem made of molybdenum

d.rotator made of cupper

e.rotation is effected by an induction motor

113. True regarding characteristic radiation

a.K_{alpha} refers to emission of a single x ray photon due to falling of electron from the L-shell to K-shell

b.K_{beta} refers to emission of a single x ray photon due to falling of electron from the L-shell to M-shell

c.L-radiation refers to radiation resulting from filling of L-shell by further outer shell

d.K radiation and L radiation has a few discrete or separate photon energies and appear as line spectrum

e.characteristic x ray energy is mainly determined by the target material but also affected by tube voltage

114. True regarding oil in x ray tube

a.oil transfer heat to housing by convection

b.housing loses heat through radiation

c.high powered tubes seen in CT and angiography may pump oil through external heat exchanger

d.the oil expand as its temperature rises

e.oil also acts as electrical insulator

115. true regarding use of stationary anode

a.intraoral (dental radiography)

b.fluoroscopy

c.mobile fluoroscopy

d.ward radiography

e. panoramic radiography(dental radiography)

116. True regarding heat rating

a.calculated in joules

b.equal to KV X m As for a constant potential or three-phase system

c.equal to 0.7 x KV_P X m As for single –phase generator

d.heat loading may be expressed in heat units

e.1.4 HU = 1 J

117.Regarding allowable m A
a.increases with effective focal spot size
b.is greater for rotating than a stationary anode
c.increase ,in rotating anode tube ,with disk diameter
d.is greater for a high speed anode
e.greater for a constant potential than a single –phase pulsating potential for exposures shorter than 1s.

118.True regarding heat rating
a.an anode heat capacity in the region of 250kj is suuficient for standard radiography
b.sufficient heat capacity in angiography may be in region of 1MJand upto 5MJ in a CT scanner
c.space charge effect refers to fact that the maximum m A is smaller at a low kv than at a kv
d.in general, X –ray tubes for diagnostic radiology donot operate above 150 kv
e.in general, the maximum m A for radiography is no greater than about 700 m A

119.True regarding characteristic radiation
a.results after ejection of the electrons from the inner orbits of the target
b.a cathode electron must have energy of more than 80 keV to eject the k shell electron of tungsten
c.In tungaten, energy of k-characteristic radiation depend on the energy of striking electrons
d.In tungsten ,energy of k-charecteristic radiation and L-characteristic radiation is about 59 keV and 11 keV respectively

e.between 80 and 150 kVp,K-shell characteristic radiation contribution is about 10-28% of useful x-ray beam

120.True regarding focal spot of x ray tube
a.focal spot refers to the area of tungsten cathode that produce the electrons
b.larger focal spot allows greater heat loading of tube
c.larger focal spot produce better radiographic detail
d.the size and shape of focal spot are determined by the size and shape of the electron stream
e.anode angle vary from 6-20^0

121.True regarding radiography
a.the subject contrast is influenced by kv
b.spatial resolution is not a function of focal spot size
c.contrast is reduced by scatter
d.unsharpness is not influenced by the focal spot size
e.unsharpness is influenced by FFD

122.True regarding x ray film.
a.polyester base (typically 0.2mm thick)
b.photographic emulsion (about 5-10 micrometer thick) ,usually on one side
c.emulsion –suspension in gelatine of silver halide crystals,generally silver iodobromide with 10%bromide and 90%iodide
d.cryastal is about 1micrometer in size and contains a million or more silver atoms
e.antistatic supercoat to protect against abrasion

123.Photographic emulsion is affected by

a.ultraviolet and visible light
b.chemical liquids and vapours
c.x rays
d.mechanical pressure and creasing
e.static electricity

124.True regarding silver iodobromide
a.small proportion of bromide relative to iodide ions distort the lattice
b.silver ions cannot move through the lattice
c.has sensitivity pecks under their surface
d.electrons accumulate at sensitivity specks
e.distribution of the specks of silver metal from the latent image

125.True regarding development of exposed x ray film
a.use of acidic solution of a reducing agent (electron donor)
b.reduce positive silver atom into silver ions
c.latent image grows into a grain of silver ions
d.bromine ions acts as barrier and repel electron donor molecules
e.the unexposed crystals usually remain unaffected by the developer

126.True regarding linear attenuation coefficient of monochromatic radiation
a.qualitative measurement of attenuation per mm of absorber
b.unit of linear attenuation coefficient is per mm
c.specific for the energy of the x ray beam
d.specific for the type of energy
e.increases with increase in the energy of radiation

127.True regarding development
of x ray film
a.background fog due to development of the unexposed crystals
b.due to penetration of developer into the the unexposed crystals
c.depend on development time
d.depend on developer strength
e.depend on developer of temperature

128.True regarding x ray tube
a.no more than 1% of electron's kinetic energy is converted into X-rays
b.$\leq$ 90 of electron's kinetic energy is converted into heat
c.cathode incorporates a fine tungsten coil or filament
d.cathode emit electrons by the process of thermionic emission at temperature like 22000 degree celsius
e.white hot cathode filament (incandescent) signify its impending breakdown

129.True regarding X- ray tube
a.a vacuum tube
b.anode ,usually of tungsten
c.electrons produced at anode
d.electrons bombard the target with a velocity of light around half the speed of light
e.positive terminal is known as cathode

130.True regarding intensifying screen
a.intensifying screen has a polyester base (typically 0.25mm) with coating of fine phosphor crystal (0.1-0.5mm)
b.intensifying screen convert the pattern of X-ray intensities into light
c.X-ray film is used only in

combination of intensifying screen
d.intraoral dental radiography uses special kind of intensifying screen
e.intensifying screen emit light of intensity inversely proportional to the intensity of the X-rays

131.True regarding phosphor used in intensifying screen
a.The absorption coefficient of the calcium tungsten is predominantly influenced by calcium
b.the absorption coefficient of calcium tungstate is not optimally matched to the typical spectra used in radiography
c.calcium tungstate emits blue light when irradiated by the X-rays
d.the sensitivity of screen should not match the spectrum of the emitted light
e.the use of calcium tungstate has been superseded by the use of rare earth materials

Answer
X- Ray tube and X-Ray production

1.bde--- X-ray tube enerygy is supplied by AC mains by means of transformer.A small increase in filament temperature produces a large increase in tube current. (page no.5/Farr)

2.ade---Single –phase ,self – rectified generator produce tube current during the positive phase of the kilovoltage cycle.It is commonly used in generator dental radiography. (page no.6/Farr)

3.abcde--Tube current refers to the number of electrons flowing /sec from the filament to the target.The number(quantity) of x rays produced depends entirely on the tube current.Electrons are produced at the filament by thermionic emission.Edison effect refers to the electron cloud surrounding the filament the connecting wires supply both the voltage (average 10v) and the amperage(average about 3-5A)
[Page 11/Christensen]

4.abcd----Distortion is reduced by using longer FFD .
(page no.57/Farr)

5.abd---Regarding x ray tube:Electron current across an x ray tube is in one direction only from the cathode to the anode.Tungsten is not more efficient than its allow for emitting electrons[Page 11-12/Christensen]

6.abc------The target angle is generally between 7-10 degree.The smaller the target angle ,the greater is the forshortening of focal spot.Use of a steeper target serves to increase the target heat rating for a given effective focal spot. (page no.59/Farr)

7.acd-----Front screen absorbs a third of the x-ray radition falling on the front screen.Intensifying screen uses fluoresroscence to erase the memory. (page no.67/Farr)

8.abcde---X- ray tube may have two or three filament,two focal spots are used in stereoscopic angiographic tube,automatic filament-boosting circuit is used to prolong tube's life,aging tubes becomes bronze-colored,vaporization alter the quality of x ray and increase possibility of arcing. [Page 13/Christensen]

9.bd---Most of energy of electrons is converted into heat,less than 1% of energy of electorns is converted into x rays.Line focus principle cause apparent decrease in focal spot size. [Page 13/Christensen]

10.abcde--Anode of x ray tube is made of tungsten and is 2-3 mm thick plate(rectangular or square,each dimension of plate >1cm)embedded in a large mass of cupper. [Page 14/Christensen]

11.abcd----Reasons for chosing Tungsten as the target material are high atomic number (74) ,so more efficient for the production of x

rays,high melting points (3370^0c),so withstand the high temperature produced,reasonably good material for the absorption of heat,reasonably good material for the rapid dissipation of the heat away from the target area.
[Page 14/Christensen]

12.cde---Increasing the tube current doesnot alter the shape of the spectrum.It increases the output of not only bremstrahlung but also of characteristic radiation also. (page no.8/Farr).

13.abcde--- (page no.8/Farr)

14.abe----Melting point of copper is 2300^0c,the actual size of target tungsten is considerably larger than the area of electron bombardment. (Page 14/Christensen)

15.abcde---- Rotating anode in x ray tube make tube capable of withastanding high generated heat by spreading the heat produced during an exposure,the diameter of the tungsten disc affects the maximum permissible loading of the anode.Rotating anode has beveled edge and it theoretically rotate at 3000 rpm.
(Page 15/ Christensen)

16.ade----In rotating anode metallic lubricant (especially silver) is used as lubricant in bearings.Heat dissipisation is by radiation through tube vacuum to the wall of tube and then into surroundings oil ant tube housing.
(Page 16/Christensen)

17.bd---In Tungsten-rhenium anode ,roughening and pitting is not a major problem.Slits or grooves in the target surface allows the material

in the focal track to expand without producing the mechanical tension.Specific gravity of molybdenum(10.2) is less than that of tungsten(19.3). (Page 16-17/Christensen)

18.abc---In Grid-controlled X-ray tube the focusing cup is used as a third electrode and it is electrically NEGATIVE relative to the filament.The voltage applied between the focusing cup and the FILAMENT act like a switch.
(Page 17-18/Christensen)

19.bde---Residual space charge exist around filament BELOW the saturation voltage because the potential applied across the tube is insufficient to cause almost all electrons to be pulled away from the filament the instant they are produced.The tube current is emission –limited /temperature limited ABOVE the saturation voltage . (Page 18/Christensen)

20.ace---Heel effect refers to variation in intensity of the x ray beam that leaves the x ray tube and is due to angling of anode leading to more intensity of x ray baem toward the cathode side of tube.The effect is less noticeable when larger focus-film distance used.(Page 18-19/Christensen)

21.abcd--- Extremely thick mineral oil between the x ray tube the housing.Because of its insulating properties .the oil allows more compact tubes and housing to be used ,because it permits points of high potential difference to be placed closer to each other.convection currents set up in the oil help to carry heat away from the tube. (Page 20/Christensen)

22.abc---The parameters that measures x-ray tube loading are the heat unit,the watt-second/joule,kilowatt rating. (Page 21/Christensen)

23.abc----Increasing the radiation energy increases the number of transmitted photons and decreases attenuation.Increasing the density,atomic number ,or electrons per gram of the absorber decreases the number of transmitted photons and increases attenuation. (Page 74-75/Christensen)

24.bcd---Maximum temperature to which tungsten can be safely raised is 3000^0c. Heat unit is defined for single phase generator. (Page 20/Christensen)

25.cde ----In the equation $N=N_0e^{-mu \times k}$, symbols ,N stands for the number of transmitted photons,N_O stands foe the number of incident photons. (Page 72/Christensen)

26.ade--- Metal/ceramic X- ray tubes contain three ceramic insulators and anode rotate on an axle. (Page 20/Christensen)

27.abc----Photons may be scattered in all directions and the electrons are projected only in sideways and forwards directions. (page no.11/Farr).

28.abcde ---Advantages of metal incasing areless off- focus radiation,longer tube life,high tube currents,higher tube loading,adequate electrical safety. (Page 25/Christensen)

29.abcd---There is more off-focus radiation in metal x ray tube than glass encased x ray tube because the the metal envelope is grounded and attract the off-focus electrons. (Page 25/Christensen)

30.abde---100 kVp means the maximum voltage across the tube is 100,000 V. (Page 29/Christensen)

31.abde--There is a wide distribution in the energy of general radiation due to different energies of striking electrons and also because the most electrons give up their energy in stages.There is a well- defined minimum wavelength of x rays produced in general radiation and this minimum wavelength (highest energy) depend on the x ray tube voltage (kVp) (minimum wavelength$=12.4/kVp$).The maximum wavelength (lowest energy) of x rays escaping the tube will depend on the filtering action of the enclosure of the x ray tube and on any added filtration. (Page 30-31/Christensen)

32.e---The ejection of Auger electrons donot produce characteristic radiation.The $alpha_1$ and $alpha_2$ characteristic x rays arise from transition of L –shell electrons to the K-shell .The $beta_1$ characteristic x rays arise from transition of M–shell electrons to the K-shell (Page 31-31/Christensen)

33.abcd---Factors affecting the intensity of the x ray beam are the kilovoltage,x ray tube current,the target material ,the filtration. (Page 33/Christensen)

34.abe---- With tungsten anode ,the x ray beam consists almost entirely of general radiation. The kVp determines the maximum energy (quality) of the x rays produced. (Page 34/Christensen)

35.abde---Tungsten has a high melting point(3370^{0C}) (Page 11/Christensen)

36.abc---

	Atomic number	melting point
tungsten	74	3370^0c
platinum	78	1770^0c
gold	79	1063^0c

(Page 34/Christensen)

37.ace---In the diagnostic energy range, x ray photons interaction is always with orbital electrons. Scatter radiation adds noise to the system . (Page 61/Christensen)

38.abc ----In coherent scattering/unmodified scattering /classical scattering, there is no energy transfer and no ionization.It produce scattered radiation and so result in film fog ,but total quantity is too small to be important for diagnostic radiology.The percentage of radiation that undergoes coherent scattering is less than 5%.(Page 62/Christensen)

39.abc---Electrons in the outermost cell are loosely bound,so its electrons are called" free electrons".the binding energy of shell is higher for the shell which is closer to the nucleus.Energy of electronic shells are also affected by the atomic number of the atom.The shell binding energy of lead is 88 keV while that of calcium is only 4 keV. (Page 62/Christensen)

40.ab----Sensitometer is used to derive characteristic curve.It has three distinct regions---the region of correct exposure,the toe and the shoulder.The toe is low-density region in which the slope of curve is shallow.The shoulder is at higher densities and also has shallow slope.The region of correct exposure is the (nearly) straight line portion,where the slope or gradient is steepest.The densities within the area of diagnostic interest should lie within this range. (page no.68/Farr).

41.ade---In photoelectric effect the incident photon disappears giving all of its energy to the electron.The photoelectric effect always produce three end products:characteristic radiation,a positive ion and a photoelectron .The photoelectron has little penetrating capacity. (Page 63/Christensen)

42.bd----induction motor rotate the anode without mechanical linkage to the rotating anode.Because of lack of direct mechanical linkage ,there is a time delay before anode comes up to its full speed of about 1ms.Anode doesnot stop immediately after static coils are de-enerzised .
(page no.60/Farr).

43.abcde----(Page 63-64/Christensen)

44. abcde----(Page 64/Christensen)

45.bcde---The photoelectric effect doesnot produce scatter radiation. (Page 65/Christensen)

46.ae---In Compton scattering,there is interaction of relatively high energy incident photons with outer shell electron,eject it as recoil electron and incident photon itsef is deflected retaining part of energy as scatter radiation. (Page 66/Christensen)

47.abcd----In Compton effect at narrow angle of deflection ,scattered photons retain almost all their original energy. (Page 67/Christensen)

48.a--- Scattered radiation with narrow angle of deflection is a serious problem in diagnostic radiology because there is a excellent chance of reaching x-ray film and producing fog,and it cannot be rmoved by filters and grids. (Page 67/Christensen)

49.abcde---- (Page 27/Christensen)

50.ad---The number of Compton reaction is indedependent of the atomic number of the absorber,the number of Compton reaction gradually decreases as photon energy increases.Compton effect is a major issue in fluoroscopy due to scatter radiation .
(Page 67-68/Christensen)

51.bcd----Due to heel effect ,there is less intensity of x rays towards the anode edge and so thicker part must be placed on cathode side. Heel effect is gradual,so not noticeable on even largest film. -(page no.62/Farr).

52.abd----Rotor is not in danger of overheating and seizing up because the molybdenum stem is sufficiently long and narrow to control the amount of heat that is conducted to rotor.The rate of heat radiation decreases as the anode assembly gets hotter,being proportional to the fourth power of

the temperature expressed in K. (page no.60/Farr).

53.abcde--- -(page no.67-68/Farr).

54.abcde---(page no.5/Farr).

 55.ab---- X- ray tubes is a diode tube containing two electrodes(cathode ,negative electrode and anode ,positive electrode. It is made of pyrex glass and is a vaccum tube.Electrons are produced at cathode and accelerated toward the anode where x rays are produced. [Page 10/Christensen]

56.bde----The wavelength of characteristic x ray doesnot depend upon the kVp.Of course the applied kilovoltage must be high enough to excite the characteristic radiation.The quality of x ray depend almost entirely on the x ray tube potential (kVp).

57.acd-- X-ray tube is a vaccum tube that allow the number and the speed of the accelerating electrons to be controlled independently.Gas in the tube produce secondary electrons .The negative terminal of the x ray tube is called the cathode.The cathode consists of filament ,connecting wires and focusing cup.The connecting wire and pyrex glass has same coefficients of linear expansion. To avod differential expansion and consequent loss of vacuum in the tube. [Page 10-11/Christensen]

58.abcde---(page no.6/Farr)

59.de---In X ray tube, electrons strikes the target with kinetic energy equivalent to half of the tube potential and penetrate several micrometers into the target.The electrons produce heat on interacting with outer electrons of the atom. (page no.6/Farr)

60.bcd----film processing use acid solution of thiosulphate ('hypo') as fixer .Washing is done to remove retained hypo and vinegary smell in the stored film may be due to retained thiosulphate. ---(page no.66/Farr)

61.abc----Optical density is measured by densitometer.The density of the area of interest on a properly exposed film averages about 1.Area with density above 3 are too dark to be viewed on a standard light box and requires a bright lamp if any detail is to be seen. (page no.66/Farr)

62.abd---The photon energy of the K radiation increases as the atomic number of target increases.The rate of production of characteristic radiation decreases as the kv increases above E_k. ---(page no.7/Farr)

63.ad---E_k of tungsten is 70 kev.Cathode emit electons.80 % or more of x ray emitted by diagnostic x ray tube are bremsstrahlung in nature

64.ac----Bremsstrahlung refrs to X rays produced by interaction of electron with the nucleus.except in mammography ,bremssstrahlung is responsible for 80% or more of the emitted xrays .The bremsstrahlung forms a continuous spectrum.The maximum photon energy (in kev) is numerically equal to tube potential (kv).there is low- energy cut off at about 20kev dur to filtarion by the target ,glass wall of the tube and other materials.---(page no.7-8/Farr)

65.abcde--- (page no.8/Farr)

66.abcde---(page no.62/Farr)

67.abd---Increasing the kv increases the effective energies of x ray photons and the efficiency of x ray production.No characteristic radiation is produced below 70kv for a tungsten target. ---(page no.8/Farr)

68.bde----Transmission ,scattering and absorption are three possible fate in interaction with matter.The x ray images is formed by the transmitted photons. ---(page no.9/Farr)

69.bc----- The half –value layer (HVL) refers to the thickness of the stated material will reduce the the intensity of x ray beam to one half of its originals .HVL=0.693 /linear attenuation coefficient.HVL can be used for beams that are not monoenergetic but applies only to narrow beams. ---(page no.9-10/Farr)

70.abcde--- ---(page no.9-10/Farr)

71.bcd---The x ray can never be completely absorbed in a material.Measured HVL would be larger in case of use of wide beam. ---(page no.9-10/Farr)

72.abcde------(page no.10/Farr)

73.bce---In Compton effect, greater the angle of scattering,the greater the energy and range of the recoil of electron.The higher the initial initial photon energy ,the greater the remaining photon energy of the scattered radiation and the greater the energy of recoil electron and its range. ---(page no.11/Farr)

74.a-------(page no.11/Farr)

75.abcde-------(page no.12/Farr)

76.d----The softening effect of Compton scatter is greatest with large scattering angles as well as with high energies X-rays.The electron density of bone ,air ,fat ,muscle and water does not vary more than 10%.The mass attenuation coefficient for the Compton effect is the same within 10% for air ,tissue ,bone,contrast media and lead.In diagnostic range ,no more than 10% of the energy is absorbed ,the rest being scattered. ---(page no.12/Farr)

77.acde---- the energy of the photon is completely absorbed in the photoelectric process---(page no.13/Farr)

78.abe ----the spectral sensitivity of the film should match the spectral emission of the screen .Calcium tungstate emits a continouous spectrum of violet and blue light. ---(page no.67/Farr)

79.abcde---- (Chapter 1,page no.13,second edition (2008),Farr's Physics for Medical Imaging).

80.acd---- Effective atomic number refers to weighted average of the atomic numbers of the constituent elements.The Compton and photoelectric interaction depend on the effective atomic number but not on the molecular configuration (Chapter 1,page no.13,second edition (2008),Farr's Physics for Medical Imaging).

81.bcde---Cassette is a flat light-tight box. ---(page no.67/Farr)

82.ce-----When the photon energy reaches E_k, the probability of photoelectric absorption jumps to a higher level (K-absorption edge).the probability of photoelectric absorption increases as photon energy increases further beyond the E_k.The higher the atomic number of the material,the greater is E_K higher the atomic number ,the greater is the photon energy at which the edge occurs.(page no.14/Farr)

83.bcd---Focusing cup surrounds the cathode and is maintained at same negative potential as that of filament.(Page 12, Christensen)

84.abcd---A material is relatively transparent to to ints own characteristic radiation because the photon energy of the K-radiation of any material is somewhat less than its E_k. (page no.14/Farr)

85.ae----The photoelectric coefficient is high when photon energy is just greater than E_k.The Compton coefficient is independent of Z(atomic number) and little affected by E.The photoelectric absorption is more important than the Compton process with high Z materials and with relatively low energy photons.The photon energy at which the photoelectric and Compton process are equally important are about 30 kev for air ,water and tissue ,50 kev for aluminium and bone ,300 kec for iodine and barium and 500 kev for lead. .(page no.14/Farr)

86.abcde----(page no.14/Farr)

87.ace---- Secondary electrons refers to recoil elecrons and photoelectrons set moving in the material by Compton and photoleclectric process, interact with outer shells of nearby atom and cause excitation and ionization ,the range is inversely proportional to the density of the material. .(page no.14-15/Farr)

88.abcde---(page no.15/Farr)

89.abcde---(page no.15/Farr)

90.abcde ---.(page no.15/Farr)

91.acde---Attenuation refers to reduction in the intensity of an x ray beam as it traverses through the matter ,not trough the x ray tube and plate. [Page 70/ Christensen]

92.ade----True regarding rare earth phosphor screen.are more efficient than calcium tungstate and more sensitive(faster) than calcium tungstate screen .Phosphors incorporate impurities that form the energy traps . [Page 70/ Christensen]

93.ade----In attenuation of monochromatic radiation,there is no reduction of quality (energies) and there is logarithmic attenuation as passes through the matter (the number of photons remaining in the beam decreases by the same percentage with each increment of absorber. [Page 71/ Christensen]

94.bce----the product of the linear attenuation coefficient and half-value layer is equal to 0.693.Beam with high half value layer is more penetrating than one with a low half value layer. [Page 73/ Christensen]

95.cde ----In the equation $N=N_0e^{-mu \times k}$, symbols ,N stands for the number of transmitted photons,N_O stands foe the number of incident photons.
[Page 72/ Christensen]

96.abc----Increasing the radiation energy increases the number of transmitted photons and decreases attenuation.Increasing the density,atomic number ,or electrons per gram of the absorber decreases the number of transmitted photons and increases attenuation. [Page 74-75/ Christensen]

97.abcde----[Page 76-77/ Christensen]

98.ade----With high atomic number absorber,transmission of radiation beam may paradoxically decrease with increasing energy.A sudden reduction in radiation transmission through lead occurs at 88keV(binding energy of the K.shell electron due to photoelectric effect.Gram for gram,Tin is better absorber of x rays then the Lead between 29-88 keV,tin attenuates more radiation per unit weight than lead.So a lighter tin apron gives the same protection as a standard lead apron. [Page 78/ Christensen]

99.abcde----[Page 79/ Christensen]

100.abcde---[Page 79/ Christensen]

101.abde---There is linear relationship between density and attenuation.if the density of a material is doubled,attenuation doubles. A difference in tissue densities is one of the primary reasons for x ray image. [Page 79/ Christensen]

102.ae----The bone has fewer electron/gram than water,lead has fewer electrons per gram than oxygen.In general ,the high atomic number elements has about 20% fewer electrons than the low atomic number elements. [Page 80/

Christensen]

103.bd----In polychromatic radiation , the energy of the most energetic photon is determined by kVp,mean energy of photons increases as low energy photons are initially eliminated during attenuation. [Page 80-81/ Christensen]

104.abcde--- The image formation depend on a differential attenuation .Greater is differential attenuation ,greater is the the contrast. [Page 81/ Christensen]

105.abcde----[Page 84/ Christensen]

106.abd---The size of the projected focal spot is directly related to the sine of the angle of the anode (anode angle).The anode angle vary from 6-20 ^{0}c .As the anode is made smaller ,the apparent focal size becomes smaller . Focal spot size is expressed of terms of the apparent focal spot ,so 0.3mm focal spot refers to its apparent size. [Page 13-14/ Christensen]

107.abc-----Geometrical unsharpness is related to the image of a stationary structure.Geometrical unsharpness is reduced by a longer FFD. (page no.57/Farr).

108.abcde---(page no.57/Farr).

109.ab---Commonly,an x ray tube has two filaments to provide two focal spots of different sizes that may be selected by the operator. The smaller focal spot is used for improved resolution and larger one for thicker parts of the body.Typical focal spot size is 0.3mm for mammography , 0.6-1.2 mm for general radiography, 0.6mm for fluoroscopy ,and 0.6-1.0mm for CT scanning.Focal spot size is not constant –depend on m A and KV. (page no.59/Farr).

110.abcde----(page no.59/Farr).

111.abcde---- (page no.57/Farr).

112.abcde---- (page no.60/Farr).

113.acd---K_{beta} refers to emission of a single x ray photon due to falling of electron from the M-shell to K-shell.Characteristic x ray energy is determined by the target material and is unaffected by tube voltage.(page no.07/Farr).

114.abcde----(page no.60/Farr).

115.abcde----(page no.60/Farr).

116.abcde----(page no.60/Farr).

117.abcde-----(page no.61/Farr).

118.abcde---- (page no.61/Farr).

119.ade---For characteristic radiation a cathode electron must have energy of more than 70 keV to eject the k shell electron of tungsten because the binding energy of an electron in the k –shell of tungsten is about 70 keV.In tungaten, the energy of k-characteristic radiation is always same regardless of the energy of striking electrons because it depend on the energy difference of k-shell and that of L or M shell.Between 80 and 150 kVp,K-shell characteristic radiation contribution is about 10-28% of useful x-ray beam.Below 70 kvP there is no k-shell characteristic radiation.Above 150kvP the contribution of characteristic radiation decreases and it becomes negligible above 300 kVp. (page no.61/Farr).

120.bde---Focal spot of x ray tube

refres to the area of tungsten target that is bombarded by electrons from the cathode ,larger focal spot allows greater heat loading of tube .smaller focal spot produce better radiographic detail,the size and shape of focal spot are determined by the size and shape of the electron stream,anode angle vary from 6-20^0[Page 13/Christensen]

121.ace----Spatial resolution is a function of focal spot size.Unsharpness is influenced by the focal spot size. (page no.65/Farr).

122.acd---X-ray film has polyester base (typically 0.2mm thick) with photographic emulsion (about 5-10 micrometer thick) ,usually on both side.Emulsion is suspension in gelatine of silver halide crystals,generally silver iodobromide with 90%bromide and 10%iodide. (page no.65/Farr).

123.abcde---(page no.65/Farr).

124.cde---In silver iodobromide ,small proportion of iodide relative to bromide ions distort the lattice.Silve ions cann move through the lattice and attacted to sensitivity specks to neutralse electrons . (page no.65/Farr).

125.de-- development of exposed x ray film is done by immerging into alkaline solution of a reducing agent (electron donor)which reduce positive silver ions into silver atoms and latent image grows into a grain of silver atoms. (page no.65/Farr).

126.cd----Linear attenuation coefficient is a quantitative measurement of attenuation per centimeter of absorber.Unit of linear attenuation coefficient is per centimeter and so it is called Linear attenuation coefficient .It decreases with increase in the energy of radiation . (page no.72/Farr).

127.abcde----(page no.72/Farr).

128.ac --->/= 99 of electron's kinetic energy is converted into heat Cathode emit electrons by the process of thermionic emission at tem like 2200 degree Celsius.white hot cathode filament (incandescent) emit electrons.

129.abe---Electrons are produced at cathode.Electrons bombard the target with a velocity around half the speed of light. ---(page no.5/Farr).

130.abc---Intraoral dental radiography uses no intensifying screen.Intensifying screen emit light of intensity proportional to the intensity of the X-rays. (page no.66/Farr).

131.bce----The absorption coefficient of the calcium tungsten is predominantly influenced by tungsten.The sensitivity of screen should match the spectrum of the emitted light. (page no.67/Farr).

CHAPTER 3
Filter ,Restrictor ,Grid ,Screen

1.True regarding grid factor

a.grid factor is defined as exposure necessary with grid /exposure necessary without a grid

b.the grid factor is typically in the range of 3-5

c.grid ratio principally depend on the grid ratio,patients thickness and KV

d.use of grid has no effect on patients dose

e.Gustav Buck y is credited with the development of the antiscatter grid

2.True regarding filtration

a.remove a large proportion of the high –energy photons before reaching the skin

b.reduce the dose received by the patient

c.refers to sheet of uniform metal ,usually aluminium(added filtration)

d.interposed between the X-ray tube and the patient

e.Compton process is predominant process involved in filtration

3.True regarding grid

a.mainly absorb primary radiation

b.mainly transmit scattered radiation

c.selectivity is judged by the fraction of primary radiation transmitted /fraction of scattered radiation transmitted

d.an upper limit of the fraction of primary radiation can be calculated from geometry of the grid

e.typically selectivity is in range of 6-12

4.True regarding filter material

a.very high atomic number

b.photoelectric process predominance

c.copper suitable for most diagnostic X rays beams

d.copper is more efficient filter than aluminium

e.copper used as compound filter with aluminium on X ray tube side

5.Effect of increasing the filtration

a.causes the continuous X- ray spectrum to shrink and move to right

b.increases the minimum and effective photon energies

c.increases the maximum photon energies

d.reduces the area of aspectum and the total output of X rays

e.decreases the exit dose:entry dose ratio or film dose :skin dose ratio

6.True regarding filtration

a.responsible for low energy cut-off of the x ray spectrum

b.K-edge filter has k-edge in lower energy part (ex.-erbium)

c.K-edge filter remove only high –energy X –rays

d.K-edge filter is relatively transparent to the energies just above the K-edge

e.K-edge filter is routinely used

7.True regarding soft or compensating or wedge filter

a.attached to x ray tube to make the exposure across the film more uniform

b.compensate for the large difference in transmission

c.used in x ray of upper and lower thorax,

d.used in x ray of neck and shoulder,or foot and ankle

e.incorporated in the beam diaphragm in fluoroscopy

8.True regarding added filtration

a.Aluminum is an excellent filter material for low energy radiation

b.Cupper is better filter than aluminum for high energy radiation.

c.almost always used filter material is copper,because it is a good general purpose filter

d.most filtration occurs in aluminum in compound filter

e.copper absorb the characteristic radiation of aluminum in compound filter

9.True regarding filter

a.recommended total filtration (inherent and added) above operating kVp of 70 is 2.5mm

b.an aluminum filter more than 3mm thickness offers no advantage

c.wedge filter is so called because of its high K –edge

d.wedge filter is often used in lower limb angiography

e.K-edge filter may be advantageous when imaging barium or iodine

10.True regarding atomic number and k-edge

a.molybdenum   42/20

b.gadolinium   64/50.2

c.holmium   67/55.6

d.iodine   53/33.17

e.barium   56/37.45

11.True statements are

a.contrast is greatest when the contrast agent absorbs x rays poorly

b.the maximum contrast is obtained when the energy of the x ray beam

is close to ,but slightly below, the k edge of the absorber

c.the purpose of K-edge filter is to produce an x ray beam that has high number of photons in specific energy range.

d.the energy spectrum transmitted by aluminum filter is too wide.

e.the gadolinium filter transmits increasing numbers of photons from the 25 to 50.2 keV range

12.True regarding filters

a.usually sheets of metal interposed between the patients and the x ray tube (added filtration)

b.reduce patients radiation dose by absorbing high energy photons

c. high inherent filtration noted in case of berrylium window

d.inherent filtarion usually varies between 0.5 mm and 1.0 mm aluminium equivalent

e.cause significant decrease of contrast   in high energy range

13.True regarding use of heavy metal filters

a.increased tube loading

b.more mAs required

c.more useful for paediatric patients

d.the holmium filter almost overlaps the region of high attenuation by iodine/barium

e.molybdenum filter used in mammography attenuate x rays just above the 20-keV

14.True regarding x –ray restrictors

b.regulate shape and size of x ray beam

c.an aperture diaphragm is made of tungsten

d.an aperture diaphragm produce less penumbra than cylinders e.cones place limitations on available field sizes

15.True regarding intensifying screen
a.the color of light emitted by the rare earth phosphor depends on the activator used
b.Turbium produces blue light
c.Two phosphor cannot be used in a single intensifying screen
d.the yttrium tantalate emit light in the ultraviolet and blue wavelengths
e.rare earth screens shows maximum speed at about 80 kVp.

16.True regarding filtration
a.target ,window ,insulating oil,the glass inert, are part of added filtration
b.inherent filtration typically equivalent to 1 mm of aluminium
c.beryllium used for added filtration
d.the amount of added is typically equivalent to 1.5mm Al
e.total filtration produce an HVL of about 2.5mm Al at 70 kv and 4.0 mm at 120 kv

17.True regarding intensification factor
a. high speed screen records more detail
b.thicker phosphor layer result in faster screen due to more absorption of x ray photons
c.fast screen and medium (par screen) has IF in range of 50,25 respectively
d.thicker phosphor layer result in decrease in clarity of image primarily due to diffusion of light
e.dye increase the speed of screen by decreasing the amount of emitted light

18.True statements are
a.x- ray film is able to record upto 100 line pairs/mm
b.cassette is not necessarily light-tight container
c.foreign material on screen produce an area of overexposure in the film
d.solution containing an antistatic compound and a detergent is used for cleaning
e.The cassette should be immediately closed after cleaning

19.True regarding collimators
a.the best general purpose beam restrictors
b.illumination of field permit accurate localization on the patients
c.provide infinite variety of rectangular x ray fields
d.enable patient radiation protection by restricting exposed field
e.less scatter radiation ,so improve film quality

20.True regarding grid ratio
a.distance between the lead strips/the height of lead strips
b.usual range is 4:1 to 16:1
c.generally higher the ratio,the better is function
d.maesure of ability to remove scatter radiation
e.second number of ratio always 1.

21.True regarding intensifying screen
a. decrease the x-ray dose to patients
b. allow use of shorter exposure time
c.use of x ray film with photo-emulsion on one side
d.no loss of information noted
e. single intensifying screen in the cassette

22.True regarding grid

a.strips are slightly angled in cross-section of focused grid

b.parallel grid has well defined convergent line

c.the focusing range is fairly narrow for a low-ratio grid

d.parallel grid is frequently used in fluoroscopic spot film devices

e.grid cassette is usually used for portable radiography

23.True regarding primary transmission(Tp)

a.Tp is measurement of the percentage of primary radiation transmitted through a grid

b.the phantom is placed at a great distance from the grid for measurement

c.T_p%=intensity with grid /intensity without grid

d.there is a insignificant loss of primary radiation with grid

e.loss of primary radiation is more with cross grid

24.True regarding development of x ray film

a.a chemical process oxidising silver ion into black metallic silver

b.amplify the latent image by a factor of millions

c.generally all or none phenomenon

d.usually initiated at the site of a latent image speck

e.time is a fundamental factor

25.True regarding the Bucky factor

a. indicates percentage of secondary radiation absorption by the grid

b.indicates increase in exposure factor on change from nongrid to grid factor

c.indicates increase of patients exposure dose on use of grid

d.Bucky factor =incident photon/transmitted photon

e.measure of grid ability to absorb secondary radiation

26.True regarding Bucky factor

a.generally high ratio grid has larger bucky factor

b.independent of energy of the x ray beam

c.high Bucky factor desirable for better film quality

d.high bucky factor increases the exposure factors

e.high Bucky factor increases patients 's radiation dose to patients

27.True regarding Contrast Improvement Factor

a.the ratio of the contrast with a grid/contrast without grid

b.the ultimate test of grid performance

c.higher the grid ratio,higher is contrast improvement factor

d.more closely related to lead content of grid than any other factor

e.relative performance of grid is dependent on kVp

28.True regarding grid cutoff

a.there is loss of primary radiation

b.due to poor geometric relationship between the primary beam and the lead foil strips of the grid

c.greater grid cutoff with low-ratio grid

d.greater grid cutoff with short grid focus distance

e.with upside down focused grid,there is no exposure in the centre of film

29.True regarding lateral decentering

a.due to x ray tube being at incorrect focal distance

b.different lead strips cutoff different amount of primary radiation

c.uniform loss of radiation over the surface of the grid

d.produce uniformly light radiograph

e.easily recognised by seeing the film

30.True regarding lateral decentering

a.the amount of cutoff increases as the grid ratio increases

b.the amount of cutoff increases as decentering distance increases

c.the amount of cutoff decreases as the focal distance increases

d.Exact centering possible in portable radiography

e.off –level grid has same effect as lateral decentering

31.True regarding combined lateral and focus-grid distance decentering

a.the most commonly recognized kind of grid cutoff is combined lateral and focus-grid distance decentering

b.causes uneven exposure to film combined lateral and focus-grid distance decentering

c.the most common type of grid cutoff is lateral decentering

d.uniformly light radiograph is produced by lateral decentering

e.dark band of exposure in the center of film is produced by upside down focused grid

32.True regarding moving grid

a.invented by Bucky in 1920,so called Bucky grid

b.used to blur out the shadows cast by the lead strips

c.single –strokes grid moves in reciprocating way

d.were important in old days due to thick strips and uneven spacing

e.transverse movement of grid synchronous with the pulses of the x-ray generator

33.True regarding grid selection

a.below 9o kVp, 8:1 grid is adequate

b.above 90 kVp, 12:1 grid is preferred

c.Crossed grid used in biplane cerebral angiography

d.there is no change in transmitted scatter between 12:1 and 16:1 ratio grid

e.crossed radiation used where there is little scatter radaion

34.True regarding air gap techniques

a.used to reduce scatter radiation

b.more x-ray exposure factors than grid?

c.more of scatter radiation miss the film

d.large quantities of radiation are absorbed in air gap

e.x ray beam is strongly hardened

35.True regarding fluorescence

a.Luminescence refers to emission of light by a substance

b.Stimuli for luminescence may be light,chemical reaction,ionizing radiation

c.In fluorescence ,light is emitted beyond 10^{-8} sec of the stimulation

d.calcium tungastate is used as phosphor in intensifying screen

e.zinc cadmium sulfide is used as phosphor in photofluorographic screen

36. True regarding grid lines

a. grid lines are shadows of the lead strips moving grid

b. superimposed on the radiological image

c. reduce definition of fine detail

d. may be seen with magnifier

e. stationary grid blur out the grid lines

37. True regarding intensifying screen

a. typical thickness ---15-16 mils

b. phosphor layer thickness reduced for high speed screen

c. titanium dioxide layer prevent damage to phosphor during cleaning

d. phosphor layer sandwitched between protctive layer and reflecting layer

e. protective layer prevent static electricity

38. True regarding air gap technique

a. no strong bias for forward scattering in the diagnostic energy range

b. ineffective technique for controlling scatter radiation in megavoltage therapy

c. most effective in removing scatter radiation when the scatter originates close to the film

d. technique used in magnification radiography and chest radiography

e. greater x ray factors than grids.

39. True regarding calcium tungstate

a. original phosphor used in x-ray intensifying screen

b. Scheelite is a natural calcium tungstate

c. absolutely free of any contaminant

for proper fluorescence

d. produce light in red region of visible spectrum

e. film sensitivity maximum to light of calcium tungstate

40. True regarding intensification factor(IF)

a. maesure of decrease of patients exposure due to use of intensifying screen

b. the ratio of the x ray exposure needed to produce the same density on a film with and without the sscreen

c. IF of calcium tungstate decreases with increase of x ray beam due to high k-edge

d. heavy filtering of x ray beam decreases IF

e. calcium tungstate IF is relatively faster in radiography of a thinner part

41. True statements regarding intensifying screen

a. The Hi plus screens is two times thick as the par screens .

b. The Hi plus screen is trice as fast as the par speed screen.

c. Yttrium is a rare earth phosphor.

d. Rare earth phosphor is also known as Lockheed phosphor.

e. thulium,terbium,gadolinium and europium are used as phosphor

42. True regarding rare earth phosphor.

a. rare earth phosphor fluoresce properly only in the pure state

b. rare earth phosphor conversion efficiency is about 20%

c. the conversion efficiency of yttrium oxysulphide screens is about the same as that of gadolinium

d. Spectral emission of Yttrium

tantalate :thulium activated is green
e.efficiency of yttrium tantalate : niobium activated phosphor is 11%

43.True regarding intensifying screen
a.the fraction of x ray beam absorbed by a pair of rare earth screens is about 60%.
b.rare earth screen develops 4-5 fold absorption advantage over calcium tungstate,in x-ray energy range of 39-70 kev.
c.K- shell binding energy of Gadolinium is 50.2 keV
d.adding Lanthanum to gadolinium screen offers no advantage.
e.yttrium is faster than calcium tungstate due to higher absorption of x ray

44.True regarding intensifying screen
a. polyester plastic used as screen support
b.reflecting coat made of titanium dioxide
c.phosphor crystals remain suspended in a plastic containing substance
d.protective layer largely composed of cellulose compound
e.reflecting layer is indispensible component of screen.

45.Intensifying agent that produce light in blue-violet range
a.Calcium tungstate (430nm)
b.Barium lead sulphate(360nm)
c.Barium strontium sulphate(360)
d.Yttrium tantalate :niobium(410)
e.gadolinium oxysulphide;terbium((544nm)

46.True regarding intensifying screen and film

a.natural silver halide screen is maximally sensitive to blue light
b.the sensitivity of natural halide film's sensitivity stops at about 500nm
c.the natural silver halide screen can be used with gadolinium oxysulphide :terbium screen
d.Gadolinium oxysulphide and Yttrium oxysulphide screens shows line emission
e.Yttrium oxysulphide screen show more speed with natural silver halide film

47.True statement
a.europium –activated-barium fluorohalide is used as photostimulable phosphor
b.Thermoluminescent dosimetry use lithium fluoride as phosphorescent material
c.Photostimulable phosphor is a material that has activator and vacancy trap
d.In BaFBr:Eu, the image is readable for up to about 8 hours at room temperature
e.helium –neon laser is used for reading photostimulable plate

48.True regarding computed radiography
a.the laser light and stimulated emission has same wavelength
b.a photostimulable phosphor have a very large dynamic range compared to film
c.the photostimulable phosphor can record exposure difference of about 10000:1
d.dynamic range of photostimulable phosphor is non linear
e.wide latitude system decrease the need for repeat exposure

49. True regarding photographic film
a. emulsion ,base ,adhesive and supercoating are components
b. emulsion usually coated on one side of base
c. supercoating protect the emulsion
d. wrinked appearance to stored x ray may be due to shrinking of base
e. original xray plates consisted of glass plate

50. True regarding film base
a. provide support for the fragile photographic emulsion
b. triacetate and polyester bases are clear and colorless
c. blue tint added to base to provide dimensional stability
d. thickness of polyester base is 7mills
e. polyeaster base is thicker than triacetate base.

51. The material used to decode the information carried by the attenuated x ray beam is
a. photographic film
b. magnetic tape
c. fluoroscopic screen
d. xerography
e. magnetic disc

52. True regarding filtration
a. 2mm of aluminum absorb nearly all photons with energies less than 20 keV
b. reduce the total number of photons in the xray beam
c. selectively removes large number of low energy photons
d. increase the mean energy of the x ray beam
e. mAs need to be decreased

53. True regarding emulsion used in photographic film
a. emulsion composed silver halide only
b. emulsion is usually coated on one side of base
c. emulsion is usually thicker than 0.5 mill
d. exact composition of emulsion is well known fact
e. most xray fil is made for use with intensifying screen

54. True regarding photographic gelatin
a. is synthesized
b. prevent clumping of silver halide grain
c. keep silver halide grain well dispersed
d. procesing solutions can cannt penetrate gelatin rapidly
e. abundant availability

55. True regarding silver halide present in photographic emulsion
a. light –sensitive material
b. 80-85 % silver bromide
c. 1-10% silver iodide
d. pure siver bromide emulsion less sensitive
e. present in crystal form in emulsion

56. True regarding intensification factor(IF)
a. maesure of decrease of patients exposure due to use of intensifying screen
b. the ratio of the x ray exposure needed to produce the same density on a film with and without the sscreen
c. IF of calcium tungstate decreases with increase of x ray beam due to high k-edge
d. heavy filtering of x ray beam decreases IF

e.calcium tungstate IF is relatively faster in radiography of a thinner part

57.True regarding silver iodobromide crystal
a.point defect due to moving out of silver ion fron normal position
b.the iodine may strain the crystal by process of dislocation
c.allylthiourea is used for chemical sensitization of a crystal
d.the sensitivity specks is made of the silver iodide
e.the sensitivity specks located inside the surface of crystal

58.True regarding process of latent image formation in x ray
a.dark area on developed radiographs is due to metallic silver
b.bromine ion release electrons on absorbing energy from light photons and itself is taken by gelatin
c.dislocation defect or an AgS sensitivity speck or silver atom act as an electron trap
d.electron gives the sensitivity speck a negative charge
e.the silver ion is neutralized by electrons to form a single silver atom

59.True regarding disadvantage of moving grids
a.costly
b.vibrate x ray table on failure
c.put limit to the minimum exposure time
d.increase patient's exposure time
e.decrease film contrast

60.True regarding latent image centers
a.clumps of silver atoms
b.site of deposit of visible metallic silver

c. theoretically at least two atoms of silver /image latent centers to be developable
d.practially minimum of three to six atoms of silver /image latent centers to be developable
e.more the silver atoms at latent image ,more the probability of grain development

61.True regarding direct x ray exposure
a.only 3-10% of the photon energy is used to produce photolytic silver
b.film sensitivity varies with the energy of x ray to the factor of 2-5
c.the film exihibit maximum photoelectric absorption of 70-kVp x rays
d.film sensitivity varies with the way of film development
e.more blackening of x ray film exposed to 50 m R (kVp-50) than to that of 50 m R(kVp-200)

62.True regarding film badge monitoring
a.based on film sensitivity to detect x ray exposure
b.metal filter in front of film
c.the accuracy of film badge monitoring of x ray exposure is +/- 20%
d.provide permanent record
e.small in size and weight

63.True regarding focus- grid distance decentering.
a.the target of x-ray tube is positioned above or below the convergent line
b.the cutoff is greater with near than with far focus-grid decentering
c.the central portion of the film is not affected
d.parallel grids have a high grid ratio

to minimise cutoff

e.serious problem arise due to far focus-grid decentering in parallel grid

64.True regarding developer

a.developing solution contain hydroquinone or phenindone or metol

b.strong alkali needed to activate hydroquinone

c.hydroquinone developer is characterized by high speed ,low contrast and fine grain

d.no synergistic effect on rate development by hydroquinone and metol

e.phenindone was discovered in 1940.

65.True regarding grids

a.invented by Dr.Gustav Bucky in 1913

b.most effective way of removing scatter radiation

c.made of cupper foil strips

d.interspace material is made of aluminum

e.scatter radiation is mostly absorbed by aluminum

66.True regarding developing solutions

a.developers reduce silver ion to metallic iron

b.contain alkali to adjust the ph and act as buffer of liberated hydrogen ion

c.contain sodium sulfite as preservative

d.contain potassium bromide as antifogant or restrainer

e.functional ph of solution is 10-11.5

67.True regarding moving grids

a.moves a short distance ,parallel to grid lines

b.movement begins before the exposure starts

c.movement stops before termination of exposure

d.moving grid is used in ward radiography

e.the Potter-Bucky grid refers to moving grid

68.True regarding K-edge filter.

a.make use of the K-absotption edge of elements with atomic number >60.

b.transmit a significantly broader spectrum of energies than aluminum

c.filtered beam has decreased number of both low and high energy photons

d.decrease the patients 's absorbed dose

e.decreases image contrast

69.True regarding intrinsic conversion efficiency of intensifying Screens

a.refers to the efficiency with which the phosphor converts x rays to light

b.refers to the ratio of the light energy liberated by the crystal to the x ray energy absorbed

c.intrinsic conversion efficiency of calcium tungstate is about 25 %

d.The new phosphor has a low conversion efficiency (up to 5%)

e.Calcium tungstate is faster than new phosphor

70.True regarding photographic gelatin

a. is synthesized

b.prevent clumping of silver halide grain

c.keep silver halide grain well

dispersed

d.procesing solutions can cannt penetrate gelatin rapidly

e.abundant availability

71.True regarding grid

a.linear grid allow the x ray tube to be angled along its length

b.crossed grid is made of two superimposed linear grids of different focusing distance

c.grid ratio of crossed grid is equal to the ratio of the two linear grids.

d. crossed grid can be used with oblique view requiring angulation of x ray tube

e.most grids are focused grid.

72.True regarding the silver iodobromide crystal

a.rhombic crystal

b.perfect crystal

c.average size 1-1.5 microns

d.6.3×10^9 crystal/cubic cm of emulsion

e.an average of 10^6-10^7 silver ion /crystal

73.True regarding development

a.developing agents and preservatives are consumed

b.bromides and acid are produced

c.oxidation reaction raises the the ph of the developer

d.oxidation reaction produce no bromide

e.replenishment rate is usually lower in low volume situation than that of high volume

74.True regarding developing solution

a.time is fundamental factor in the developing process

b.coloreless meterials is produced by developing agents

c.sulfite act as a preservative by

decrease the rate of oxidation of hydroquinone

d.the significant difference in commercial x ray developing solution is in antifoggants

e.hydroquinone concentration limits the life of developing solution

75.True regarding fixing

a.removes silver halide that has not been reduced

b.silver bromide is slightly soluble in water

c.thiosulphate is used as fixer

d.a chromium or aluminium compound is used to harden gelatin

e.incompletly fixed fil appears milky

76.True regarding grid

a.made of lead

b.gap is filled with aluminium /carbon fibre

c.the line density is generally in the range of 30-40

d.the grid ratio is the ratio of the depth of the interspace channel divided by its width

e.grid required in air gap technique

77.True regarding grid

a.the larger the grid ratio, the larger is the angle of acceptance

b. the larger the grid ratio,more efficient at absorbing scatterd radiation

c. the larger the grid ratio,the greater is the contrast in the image

d.high grid ratio(12:1 or 16:1) is preferable in large fields ,especially at high KV

e.contrast imporovement factor is typically 2 and 4

78.True regarding grids.

a.unfocussed grid has parallel lead strips

b.complete cut-off noted in

unfocussed grid when the x ray beam strike at an angle that is half the acceptance angle

c.lead strips are are tilted pointing away from the tube focus in focused grid

d.there is no effect on grid cut off when focused grid is placed upside down

e.the focused grid must be used at a specific distance from the anode.

79.True regarding effect of filtration

a.attenuates the lower - energy X-rays more in proportion than the higher energy x rays

b.increases the penetrating (HVL) of the beam

c.increases intensity of x-ray beam

d.reduces skin dose to patients

e. dramatic effect over the radiological image

80.True regarding intensifying screen

a.lanthanum oxybromide ,activated with terbium ,emits a line spectrum of red light

b. lanthanum oxybromide ,activated with terbium can be used with ordinary X-ray

c.Gadolinium and lanthanum oxysulphide activated with terbium emit yollow light

d. Gadolinium and lanthanum oxysulphide activated with terbium can be used with an orthochromatic film

e.red safe light is necessary in orthochromatic film while amber safe light is used with ordinary x ray film

Answer
Filter ,Restrictor ,Grid ,Screen

1.abce--- use of grid increases patients dose. (page no.56/Farr).

2.bcd----- Filtration remove a large proportion of the low–energy photons before reaching the skin .Photoelectric process is predominant process involved in filtration. (page no.15/Farr).

3.cde----True regarding grid mainly transmit primary radiation and mainly mainly absorb scattered radiation.
(page no.56/Farr).

4.bd---Filter material should have sufficiently high atomic number to make the photoelectric process predominant interaction .Aluminium is suitable suitable for most diagnostic X rays beams(atomic number =13,E_k=1.6 kev). copper used as compound filter with aluminium on patients side because copper emits 9kev characteristic X rays .(page no.16/Farr).

5.abd---- Increasing the filtration doesnot affect the maximum photon energies and increases the exit dose:entry dose ratio or film dose :skin dose ratio
(page no.16/Farr).

6.ad----K-edge filter has k-edge in higher energy part (ex.-erbium---atomic number =68,E_k=57ekv).K-edge filter remove both high and low-energy X –rays K-edge filter is relatively transparent to the energies just above the K-edge.K-edge filter

rarely used except in mammography. (page no.16/Farr).

7.abcde----(Chapter 1,page no.16,second edition (page no./Farr).

8.ab----Aluminum is an excellent filter material for low energy radiation and a good general purpose filter . Copper is never used by itself as the filter material .It is always used in combination with aluminum as a compound filter where the copper faces the x ray tube and aluminum faces the patients.Most filtration occurs in copper in compound filter.Aluminum absorb the characteristic radiation of copper(8keV) .
[Page 88/ Christensen]

9.abde---Wedge filter is so called because of its shape.
[Page 88-90/ Christensen]

10.abcde--- [Page 90/ Christensen]

11.cde----Contrast is greatest when the contrast agent absorbs x rays most efficiently.The maximum contrast is obtained when the energy of the x ray beam is close to ,but slightly above, the k edge of the absorber.
[Page 90-91/ Christensen]

12.acd---Filters reduce patients radiation dose by absorbing low energy photons. Berrylium window is used to produce unfiltered beam .The filters increase the mean energy of an x-ray beam ,so decreases tissue contrast ,but is significant in only case of low energy radiation range. [Page 87/ Christensen]

13.abcde— [Page 91-92/ Christensen]

14.abd---An aperture diaphragm is made of sheet of lead with ahloe in middle. aperture diaphragm produce more penumbra than cylinders.
[Page 93/ Christensen]

15.ade-----Turbium produces green light while thulium produces blue light.Two phosphor can be used in a single intensifying screen which allows wider choice of film. [Page 129-31/ Christensen]

16.bde----- a.target ,window ,insulating oil,the glass inert, are part of inherent filtration .The light bbeam diaphragm mirror and the dose area product are also its part.Beryllium window used for minimizing inherent filtration filtration. (page no.15/Farr).

17.bd-----The speed of a calcium tungstate screen and its ability to record detail are in reciprocal relationship ,that is ,high speed screen records less detail.Fast screen ,medium (par screen) and slow screen (detail) has IF in range of100, 50,25 respectively.Dye decrease the speed of screen by decreasing the amount of emitted light . [Page 123-23/ Christensen]

18.ad-----Cassette is necessarily light- tight container.Foreign material on screen produce an area of underexposure in the film.The cassette should never be closed after cleaning until it is absolutely dry. [Page 123-124/ Christensen]

19.abcde---- [Page 88/ Christensen]

20.bcde----Grid ratio is a ratio of the height of lead strips /distance between the lead strips. [Page 99/Christensen]

21.ab---- the x ray film used with intensifyinfg screen has photosensitive emulsion on both sides The film is sandwitched between two intensifying screens in a cassette.The transfer of information from x ray beam to screen to film results in some loss of information. [Page 118/ Christensen]

22.ade----Strips are slightly angled in cross-section of focused grid whereas it is parallel in parallel grid.Parallel grid are focused at infinity ,so they donot have of a convergent line.the convergent line is noted in linear focused grid .the convergent point is noted in crossed grid.The focusing range is fairly wide and narrow for a high –ratio grid. [Page 100/ Christensen]

23.abc----In primary transmission(Tp),there is a significant loss of primary radiation with grid and loss of primary radiation is less with cross grid. [Page 101-102/ Christensen]

24.bcde---Development of x ray film is a chemical process reducing silver ion into black metallic silver.The developer is a reducing agent .[Page 143/ Christensen]

25.abcde ---- [Page 103-104/ Christensen]

26.acde----The size of Bucky factor depends on of energy of the x ray beam.For example ,Bucky factor for the 16:1 increases from

4.5 to 6 as the radiation increases energy increases from 70 to 120 kVp.[Page 104/ Christensen]

27.abcd---Relative performance of grid is independent on kVp,field size and part thickness.the grid which perform better at low energy radiation also performs better at high energy radiation.
[Page 104/ Christensen]

28.abd---There is a greater grid cutoff with high-ratio grid.With upside down focused grid ,there is severe peripheral cutoff with a dark band of exposure in the center of the film and no exposure at the film 's periphery .the higher the grid ratio,the narrower the exposed area.
[Page 106/ Christensen]

29.cd----Lateral decentering is probably the most common kind of grid cutoff.It results from the x-ray tube being positioned lateral to the convergent line but at the correct focal distance.All the lead strips cut off same amount of primary radiation.The center and both edges of the film are equally exposed ,and it is impossible to recognize the cutoff from inspection of the film.Cutoff increases in amount with increasing lateral decentering.
[Page 106/ Christensen]

30.abce----Exact centering is not possible in portable radiography ,low-ratio grids and long focal distances should be used whenever possible. [Page 107-108/ Christensen]

31.abcde---- [Page 109-10/ Christensen]

 32.bde----Moving grid was invented by Dr. Hollis E. Potter in 1920. Single –stroke grid moves in one direction only .Most of grid moves in reciprocating way ,which means they move continuously 1 to 3 cm back and forth throught exposure.To avoid grid lines by moving grid ,grid must move fast enough and its transverse motion should be synchronous with the pulses of the x- ray generator.[Page 110-11/ Christensen]

33.abcd---Crossed radiation is used where there is a great deal of scatter radaion,so used in biplane cerebral angiography.[Page 112/ Christensen]

34.abc----Negligible quantities of radiation are absorbed in air gap and the xray is not appreciably hardened.
[Page 112/ Christensen]

35.abde---In fluorescence ,light is emitted within 10^{-8} sec of the stimulation.In phosphorescence ,light emission is delayed beyond 10^{-8} sec of the stimulation.
[Page 118/ Christensen]

36.bcd----Grid lines are shadows of the lead strips of stationary grid superimposed on the radiological image.Moving grid blur out the grid lines. [Page 56/ Christensen]

37.ade ---- Phosphor layer thickness is increased 1-2 mils in high speed screen,and decreased slightly in detail screen.the thickness of the phosphor layer is about 4 mils forpar speed screen.Protective layer layer prevent damage to phosphor during cleaning,helps to prevent static electricity and gives physical protection to the delicate phosphor layer. [Page 119/

Christensen]

38.abcde-----Air gap technique is ineffective technique for controlling scatter radiation in megavoltage as there is strong forward bias of scatter radiation in high energy range .[Page 112-113/ Christensen]

39.abce-----Calcium tungstate produce light primarily in the blue region of the visible spectrum.Although the eye is not sensitive to light of this wavelength ,x ray emulsion exhibits maximum sensitivity to light from calcium tungstate. [Page 119/ Christensen]

40.ab----- Intensification factor(IF) of calcium tungstate increases with increase of x ray beam due to high k-edge.Heavy filtering of x ray beam increases IF.Calcium tungstate IF is relatively faster in radiography of a thicker part.[Page 121/ Christensen]

41.de----Increasing the phosphor thickness is a major way in which the speed of calcium tungstate screens is increased.The Hi plus screen is twice as fast as the par speed screen because Hi plus screen absorbs(40% of x ray beam) about twice to that of the par speed screen(20%).The Hi plus screens is not two times thick as the par screens rather they are about 2.3 times as thick as the par screens.Yttrium is not a rare earth phosphor. [Page 124/ Christensen]

42.bce---Rare earth phosphor donot fluoresce properly only in the pure state unlike calcium tungstate Spectral emission of Yttrium tantalate :thulium activated is ultraviolet /blue light.Gadolinium oxysulphide emit blue light.

[Page 125/ Christensen]

43.ac----Rare earth screen (Gd)develops 4-5 fold absorption advantage over calcium tungstate in x-ray energy range of 50-70 kev because K- shell binding energy of gadolinium is 50.2 keV.Adding Lanthanum (k-edge---38.2)to gadolinium screen offers significant absorption advantage over calcium tungstate in the 39-70-keV range.The absorption of Yttrium is the same as that of tungsten from 17-70keV ,but yttrium is faster than calcium tungstate due to higher conversion efficiency(11% vs 5%) .[Page 126-127/ Christensen]

44.acd—Some intensifying screen does not have reflecting layer ,so it reflecting layer is not indispensible component of screen.Reflecting coat is made of white substance (titanium dioxide) [Page 119/ Christensen]

45.abcd----- Gadolinium oxysulphide;terbium(544nm) intensifying agent produces light in green range [Page 128/ Christensen]

46.abd---The sensitivity of natural halide film's sensitivity stops at about 500nm, the natural silver halide screen cannot be used with gadolinium oxysulphide :terbium screen(green emission). A large fraction of the emission from yttrium oxysulphide fall within the sensitivity of natural silver halide films,so it can be used with natural halide film but yttrium oxysulphide screen show more speed with green sensitive film .[Page 129/ Christensen]

47.abcde— [Page 133/

Christensen]

48.bce---The laser light and stimulated emission has different wavelength.Dynamic range of photostimulable phosphor is linear. [Page 133-35/ Christensen]

49.acde---- Emulsion is usually coated on both sides of x ray film base [Chapter 10,Page 137-38, 4th edi77.True regarding filtration [Page 88-89/ Christensen]

50.abd----Blue tint added to base is easier to look at and produce less strain. Polyeaster base(7mills) is thinner than triacetate base(8mills)[Page 138/ Christensen]

51.abcde---- [Page 137/ Christensen]

52.abcd----The major disadvantage of filtration is reduction in the intensity of the x ray beam ,so mAs need to be increased to compensate . [Page 88-89/ Christensen]

53.de---Photographic film emulsion is composed of gelatin and silver halide.Emulsion is usually coated on both side of base.Emulsion is usually no thicker than 0.5 mill.[Page 138-39/ Christensen]

54.bce--- Photographic gelatin is made from bone .Procesing solutions can penetrate gelatin rapidly without destroying its strength or permanence. .[Page 139/ Christensen]

55.acde--- Silver halide present in photographic emulsion consists of 90-99 % silver bromide.[Page 139/ Christensen]

56.ab----- Intensification factor(IF) of calcium tungstate increases with increase of x ray beam due to high k-edge.Heavy filtering of x ray beam

increases IF.Calcium tungstate IF is relatively faster in radiography of thicker part.[Page 121/ Christensen]

57.abc-----Allylthiourea is used for chemical sensitization of a crystal,so the sensitivity specks is made of the silver sulphide .The sensitivity specks is located on the surface of crystal.It is sensitivity specks that traps electrons to begin formation of the latent image centers. [Page 139-40/ Christensen]

58.abcde---- [Page 140/ Christensen]

59.abcd---Moving grids increase the film contrast. [Page 111/ Christensen]

60.abcde----[Page 140-41/ Christensen]

61.ade---In direct x ray exposure,film sensitivity varies with the energy of x ray to the factor of 20-50..The film exihibit maximum photoelectric absorption of 50-kVp x rays because average energy of such x ray is near about k-edge of silver(25.5 keV) and bromine (13.5 keV) [Page 142/ Christensen]

62.abcde----In film badge monitoring, metal filter is used to control the energy of x rays that reaches to different areas of the film. [Page 142/ Christensen]

63.abc----Parallel grids usually have a low grid ratio to minimise cutoff.Parallel grids are focused at infinity ,so they are always used with near grid focus distance decentering.A film taken with a parallel grid has a dark center and light edges of near focus-grid distance decentering.[Page 109/ Christensen]

64.b----Developing solution contain two agents hydroquinone and phenindone or metol because of synergistic effect on rate of development .Hydroquinone is characterised by high contrast while metol developer is characterized by high speed ,low contrast and fine grain.Phenindone was discovered in 1940,metol in 1891 1md hydroquinone in 1880.[Page 143/ Christensen]

65.abd---- Grids are made of lead foil strips seprated by x-ray transparent interspacers (aluminium or some organic compound. The main function of the interspace material is to support the thin lead foil strips. [Page 99/ Christensen]

66.abcde--- [Page 143/ Christensen]

67.be----Moving grid moves a short distance ,perpendicular to to grid lines.It may move a fixed distance from side to side ,with damped oscillation or in a single movement with speed reducing with exposure time.Movement of grid does not stop moving ntil after the exposure has terminated. Stationary grid is used in ward radiography.Stationary grid used with digital imaging system such as computed radiography or direct digital radiography can produce interference patterns on the image. [Page 56/ Christensen]

68.acd--- K-edge filter (heavy metal filters) transmit a significantly narrower spectrum of energies than aluminum.It increases image contrast by reduction in high energy photons (so,more photoelectric and less Compton attenuation) [Page 90-91/ Christensen]

69.ab----Intrinsic conversion efficiency of calcium tungstate is about 5%.The new phosphor has high conversion efficiency (up to 50%).New phospher is faster than calcium tungstate.[Page 120/ Christensen]

70.bce--- Photographic gelatin is made from bone .Procesing solutions can penetrate gelatin rapidly without destroying its strength or permanence. [Page 139/ Christensen]

71.ace---Crossed grid is made of two superimposed linear grids of same focusing distance,crossed grid cannot be used with oblique view requiring angulation of x ray tube. [Page 100/ Christensen]

72.cde------ The silver iodobromide crystal is cubic in nature and it is not a perfect crystal because perfect crystal has almost no photographic sensitivity [Page 139/ Christensen]

73.abcd----Replenishment rate is usually higher(about 90 ml/14 x 17 inch film) in low volume situation than that of high volume.[Page 145/ Christensen]

74.acd-----the oxidation products of the developing agents decompose in alkaline solution and form colored materials that can stain the emulsion..these meterials reacts rapdly with sodium sulfite to form colorless soluble sulfonates .It is increase in bromide concentration that limits the life of developing solutions. [Page 143-44/ Christensen]

75.abcde----[Page 145/ Christensen]

76.abcd----Grid is not required in air gap technique.It is not used with thin parts of the body such as extrimities or with children because less scatter is generated in the patients.[Page 55/ Christensen]

77.bcde----The larger the grid ratio, the smaller is the angle of acceptance. [Page 55-56/ Christensen]

78.abe-----Lead strips are are tilted pointing toward the tube focus in focused grid.there is dramatic effect on grid cut off when focused grid is placed upside down. [Page 56/ Christensen]

79.abd---- filtration reduces intensity of x-ray beam and has little effect on radiological image.[Page 16/ Christensen]

80.bde----Lanthanum oxybromide ,activated with terbium ,emits a line spectrum of blue light lanthanum oxysulphide activated with terbium emit green light. [Page 67/ Christensen]

CHAPTER 4
Fluoroscopy

1.True regarding fluoroscopy

a.a sequence of images is viewed in real time

b.direct viewing fluoroscopy involved the use of zinc sulphide fluorescent screens

c.the brightness of the image in direct viewing fluoroscopy is very dim

d. direct viewing fluoroscopy doesnot need dark room

e.the development of the image intensifier dates back to the 1950s and 1960s

2.True regading vision

a.rod is more sensitive than cone

b.a contrast difference of 2% would be probably detectable at a light intensity of 100 millilambert (typical viewing conditions)

c.the minimum detectable sepration between two objects viewed from about 25 cm is better than 1 mm in cone vision

d.there is the need for dark adaptation (upto 30 min) in rod vision

e.there is loss color sensitivity in rod

3.True regarding scotopic vision

a.rods functions best with low levels of illumination

b.maximum concentration of rods at the fovea

c.fluoroscopy needs rod vision

d.rods are most sensitive to red region

e.use of red goggles over 30 minutes for dark adaptation

4.True regarding cesium iodide screen

a.peak energy of x ray beam in most fluoroscopy is 80 to 120kVp

b.mean energy of xray beam in most fluoroscopy is 60 kVp

c.The K-edge of cesium is 36 kev

d.absorb approximately one third of of the incident beam

e.cesium iodide phoshphor thickness one third of zinc-cadmium sulphide screen

5.True regarding photocathode used in image intensifier

a.photoabsorptive metal

b.combination of antimony and cesium compound

c.photocathode emit photopositron

d.applied directly to the CsI phosphor

e.photopositron emitted directly proportional to intensity of light

6.True regarding digital substraction angiography

a.produce images of contrast-filled vessels in isolation from other tissues

b.lead to improved clarity in the image of the vessels

c.permits use of lower dose of contrast medium

d.images of the same region are taken before and after injection of contrast medium e.avoid any movement of the patient or equipment and so images generally acquired in rapid succession

7.True regarding image intensifier

a.lens used is made of pyrex
b.lens inverts and reverses the image(point inversion)
c.the input surface is perfectly flat
d.the anode is located in the neck of the image tube
e.the anode has a positive potential of 25 to 35 Kv relative to the photocathode

8.True regarding output phosphor

a.silver activated zinc cadmium sulphide used as output phosphor
b.diameter in most output screen – 1/2 to 1 inch
c.no of light photons increased about 50-fold
d.thin layer of aluminium prevent retrograde low of light
e.closed circuit television chain used to view the output image

9.True regarding brightness gain (intensification factor)

a.use of Patterson B-2 fluoroscopic screen to compare
b. the conversion factor--- luminance of the output phosphor/the input exposure rate
c.the conversion factor usually equals about 1% of the brightness gain
d. brightness gain tends to deteriorate as an image intensifier ages
e.brightness gain==minification gain x flux gain

10.True regarding image quality in fluoroscopy

a.spatial resolution is principally limited by blurring caused by the spread of light in the output phosphor
b.spatial resolution on display monitor is no better than about 1.2 lp mm^{-1}
c.the quantum sink corresponds to the photons absorbed in the input screen
d.noise may be reduced by increasing the input dose rate and by frame averaging
e.veiling glare reduce image contrast

11.True regarding minification gain and flux gain

a.mininfication gain =(diameter of input screen)^2/(diameter of output screen)^2
b.minification improve the statistical quality of the fluoroscopic image
c.through minification, brightness can be theoretically increased indefinitely
d.flux gain increase brightness by a factor of 50
e.most image intensifier has input screen of 5 to 9 inch.

12. True regarding image intensifier design

a.the input fluorescent screen absorbs x rays and convert into light
b.photocathode emit electrons
c.high potential difference between photocathode and the accelerating anode
d.electrostatic lens guides electrons to output fluorescent screen
e.output screen emits light photons that carry the fluoroscopic image

13.True regarding image

characteristics of image intensifier

a.transmitted photons to output screen and retrograde light from the output screen reduce contrast

b.lag refers to persistence of luminescence after x ray stimulation has been terminated.

c.with CsI tubes ,lag timers are about 1ms

d.peripheral distortion(pincushion effect) due flaring of central electrons from the ideal course

e.vignetting refers to a fall-off in brightness at the periphery of image

14.True regarding image intensifier

a.the center og image has better resolution ,a brighter image and less geometric distiortion

b.field size is changed by electronic principle

c.the physical size of the input and output screens is the same in the 6-inch and 9-inch modes

d.A 9-inch omage intensifier encompass 9-inch field in the patients.

e.large field of view image intensifier tubes have an all metal envelope

15.True regarding the image intensifier

a.has inert gas filled glass or ceramic envelope

b.metal housing shield the device from the effects of magnetic effect

c.the input screen radius of curvature is approx.half of the distance from the screen to the focal point of the electron beam

d.phosphor material is antimony caesium

e.the photocathode used is caesium iodide

16.True regarding input screen

a.input phosphor layer is inner side of metal layer

b.photocathode produce light in proportion to the intensity of X-ray photons

c.the input screen is maintained at a high positive voltage with respect to the anode (difference of about 25kv)

d.the input screen size may be between about 150 and 400 mm in diameter

e.electrons are accelerated towards the anode

17.True regarding caesium iodide

a.K-edge of caesium is 36 KeV while K-edge of iodine is 33 KeV

b.about 60% of incoming X –ray photons are detected by 0.1 to 0.4 mm thick the phosphor layer

c.has norrow needle-like crystal (approx. 5 micrometer)

d.cryatal laid down perpendicular to the screen

e.crystal orientation in the phosphor promote unsharpness

18.True regarding output screen of fluoroscopy

a.size about 25 to 35 mm, few micrometers in thickness

b.caesium iodide is used as phosphor converting electron intensities into light

c.front of the screen is covered with about 0.5mm aluminium

d.aluminium coats prevent emitted light to reach photocathode

e.aluminium coats acts as cathode

19.True regarding image intensifier

a.flux gain is typically about 50
b.flux gain is due to emission of many light photons from the input phosphor by single electron
c.minification gain refers to intensification
d.minification gain is equal to the ratio of the areas of the two screens
e.the overall brightness gain is the product of the flux gain and minification gain

20.True regarding image intensifier
a.gain is a measurable quantity
b.conversion factor defines the performance of an image intensifier
c.conversion factor is defined as the ratio of the brightness (luminence) of the output phosphor and the dose rate at the input surface of the image intensifier
d.typical values of conversion factor is in the range of 250-300 Cd m^{-2}
e.gain and so conversion factor deteriorates in time and with equipment usage

21.True regarding magnification mode of image intensifier
a.the electron crossover is moved nearer to the output screen
b.effectively reduces the minification gain so reduced brightness at output screen
c.increase in exposure needed to restore brightness
d.at least one magnified field of view in all image intensifier systems
e.change of the voltages of the intermediate electrodes done for magnification

22.True regarding image intensifier system
a.lens system used in original TV

image intensifier system to focus the image on input screen of the camera
b.the signal from the video camera is converted to analog format in digital fluoroscopy
c.TV camera are standard for image intensifier-based fluoroscopy systems
d.CCDs cameras has the smaller dynamic range
e.processing of image can be done in real time in digital fluoroscopy

23.Image- processing functions in digital fluoroscopy is /are
a.noise reduction
b.edge enhancement
c.black and white reversal
d.geometrical inversion
e.mapping

24.True regarding fluoroscopy
a.automatic brightness control is not essential
b. the light intensity of the output screen is used as input signal for automatic brightness control
c.the signal from the camera is used as input signal for automatic brightness control
d.adjustment of brightness is made by increasing either kV or Ma or both
e.the area of the output screen used by the ABC system is full screen

25.True regarding fluoroscopy dose rates
a.dose rate depend on the detective quantum efficiency
b.the critical factor in determining dose rate is the level of noise
c.the lower the input dose rate to the intensifier ,the lesser is the noise in the displayed image
d.the systems with low output dose

rates will generally have lower ESD(entrance surface dose)

e.typical ESD rates is in range of 10-30 mGy min^{-1}

26. True regarding fluorography

a.a term used for recording images produced by an image intensifier

b.last image hold refers to last frame of a fluoroscopy sequence that continued to be displayed after X-ray beam has been switched off

c.fluoro grab refers to image stored permanently as record or for subsequent reporting

d.digital spot image is taken at a high m A

e.digital spot image generally require an image intensifier dose in the range of 0.1-5 micro Gy

27. True regarding veiling glare

a.smaller the image intensifier, the greater is the veiling glare

b.caused by light scattering in the output window of the intensifier

c.main cause is X-ray and light scattering in the input phosphor

d.caused by electron scattering in the tube

e.cause vignetting

28. True regarding testing image quality in fluoroscopy

a.contrast resolution is tested using a grid test object

b.a low kv is used to minimize scatter to test spatial resolution

c.grid test detect any deterioration in the focusing of the image intensifier

d.spatial resolution may be tested with a low-contrast test object

e.Leed test objects are meant for testing contrast resolution

29. True regarding the image intensifier

a.The system has yamma=0.5

b.the gamma of image intensifier is similar to a film-screen radiography

c.the focusing electrode at positive energies act as an electron lens

d.the pattern of electron intensities falling on the screen are an exact (but minified) replica of the pattern of intensities on the input screen

e.gain is the ratio of the brightness of the output phosphor to that of the input phosphor

30. True regarding magnification mode of image intensifier

a.the electron crossover is moved nearer to the output screen

b.effectively reduces the minification gain so reduced brightness at output screen

c.increase in exposure needed to restore brightness

d.at least one magnified field of view in all image intensifier systems

e.change of the voltages of the intermediate electrodes done for magnification

31. True regarding Leed tests T0.10

a.used to assess low-contrast resolution

b.It incorporates 12 groups of circular details

c.each group comprises nine disks with thickness varying progressively

d.the system is used to test fluoroscopy images using 1-2 mm of cupper filtration

e.generally not possible to see more than about six details in each group

32. True regarding flat plate detectors used in fluoroscopy

a.use amorphous silicon detectors

with caesium iodide scintillators
b.DQE is comparable to that of image intensifier (about 65%)
c.has increased dynamic range and improved spatial resolution
d.high contrast resolution (3lp mm⁻¹)
e.no distortion in the displayed image

33.True regarding advantages of cesium iodide over zinc cadmium sulphide as input fluorescent screen
a.greater packing density
b.more favorable effective atomic number
c.thinner phosphor layer (0.1mm)
d.improved resolution(3 to 5lp/mm)
e.improved image quality

34.True regarding input phosphor
a.Cesium iodide used as input fluorescent
b.use of vapor deposition process to deposit input fluorescent
c.rhombic- shaped crystal of fluorescent perpendicular to the aluminum substrate
d.abundant diffusion of light produced by phosphor layer
e.older image intensifier uses zinc cadmium sulphide screen

35.True regarding the DSA
a.the mask image refers to non-contrast image stored in the computer memory
b.mask image shows normal anatomy only
c.the mask image is substracted from the contrast image on a pixel by pixel basis
d.in general ,the substracted image

be viewed in real time
e.pixel shifting minimize the effect of movement between frames

36.True regarding digital substraction angiography
a.prior to substraction ,the contrast images and the mask are converted into logarithms
b.adding of successive frames improves the signal to noise ratio
c.the substracted image appears less noisier
d.several mask images acquired in femoral angiography
e.rotational angiography permits identification of the optimum imaging angle to view vessels

37.True regarding dual energy substraction
a.images taken in rapid succession at low and high kV
b.at high KV ,the contrast of bone is significantly improved
c.substracting the low kv image from the high kv image decreases soft tissue contrast
d. substracting the high kv image from the low kv image displays the bony structures in greater detail
e.there is no role of dual energy substraction in chest radiography.

38.True regarding pulsed fluoroscopy
a.dose rate falls approximatetely in proportion to pulse rate
b. flickering is seen in static scene at lower pulse rate
c.in grid-controlled fluoroscopy ,an additional electrode is built into the tube between the cathode and anode
d.the switching is less precise in grid controlled fluoroscopy

e.greater control over the intensity of the X- ray beam in each pulse in grid controlled fluoroscopy

39.True regarding dose control curves

a.brightness curves programmed into the system by the manufacturer

b.most generators have several dose control programmes

c.anti-isowatt curve has a lower m A at each kv setting

d.a high KV curve is suitable for paediatrics

e.automatic brightness control is achieved by feedback mechanism

40.True regarding scotopic vision

a.rods functions best with low levels of illumination

b.maximum concentration of rods at the fovea

c.fluoroscopy needs rod vision

d.rods are most sensitive to red region

e.use of red goggles over 30 minutes for dark adaptation

41.True regarding automatic brightness control

a.automatic brightness control is not essential

b. the light intensity of the output screen is used as input signal for automatic brightness control

c.the signal from the camera is used as input signal for automatic brightness control

d.adjustment of brightness is made by increasing either kV or Ma or both

e.the area of the output screen used by the ABC system is full screen

42.True regarding fluoroscopy dose rates

a.dose rate depend on the detective quantum efficiency

b.the critical factor in determining dose rate is the level of noise

c.the lower the input dose rate to the intensifier ,the lesser is the noise in the displayed image

d.the systems with low output dose rates will generally have lower ESD(entrance surface dose)

e.typical ESD rates is in range of 10-30 mGy min^{-1}

Answer

Fluoroscopy

1.abce----Direct viewing fluoroscopy need dark room. .(page no.91/Farr).

2.abcde----(page 193-94/P Dendy)

3.ace----Maximum concentration of rods is in the periphery of retin.Rods are most sensitive to ble-green light. [Page 166/ Christensen].

4.ace---- the mean energy of an x ray beam is approximately one third of its peak energy .The peak energy of x ray beam in most fluoroscopy is 80 to 120kVp,so its mean energy of x ray beam in most fluoroscopy is 30 to 40 kVp.The cesium iodide absorb approximately two third of of the incident beam. [Page 167-68/ Christensen].

5.bd----Photocathode is a photoabsorptive metal(combination of antimony and cesium compound) and emit photoelectron directly proportional to intensity of light. [Page 68/ Christensen].

6.abcde---(page no.99/Farr).

7.bde----In image intensifier,lens used is made of a series of positively charged electrodes that are usually plated onto the inside surface of the glass envelope .The input phosphor is curved to ensure that electrons emitted at the peripheral regions of the photocathode travel the same distance as those emitted from the central region. [Page 168/ Christensen].

8.abcde----[Page 169/ Christensen].

9.abcde---- [Page 170-71/ Christensen].

10.abcde----[Page 98/ Christensen].

11.abcde—[Page 171/ Christensen].

12.abcde---Image intensifier is a vaccum tube containing four basic components---1.input phosphor and photocathode 2.electrostatic focusing lens 3.accelerating anode 4.output phosphor.[Page 166/ Christensen].

13.abcde-----[Page 172-73/ Christensen].

14.abcde---[Page 172-73/ Christensen].

15.b----The image intensifier has evacuated glass or ceramic envelope .The input screen radius of curvature is approx.equal to the distance from the screen to the focal point of the electron beam.Photocathode material is antimony caesium.The phosphor used is caesium iodide. [Page 92/ Christensen].

16.bde---Input phosphor layer is on x ray beam side of metal layer.The input screen is maintained at a high negative voltage with respect to the anode (difference of about 25kv).

74

(page no.92/Farr).

17.abcd---- Caesium iodide crystal orientation in the phosphor minimizes unsharpness .Here perpendicular orientation of cryatal minimizes the spread of light in the phosphor light. (page no.92/Farr).

18.ade---In output screen, zinc cadmium sulphide is used as phosphor converting electron intensities into light and back of the screen is covered with about 0.5mm aluminium. (page no.93/Farr).

19.abcde---(page no.93/Farr).

20.bce--- Gain is a not a measurable quantity. Typical values of conversion factor is in the range of 25-30 Cd m^{-2}(page no.93/Farr).

21.bcde---- Change of the voltages of the intermediate electrodes lead to magnification mode of image intensifier .The electron crossover is moved nearer to the input screen. (page no.93/Farr).

22.ae----The signal from the video camera is converted to digital format in digital fluoroscopy.CCDs are standard for image intensifier-based fluoroscopy systems.CCDs cameras has the increased dynamic range because CCD cameras generally have 12-bit image depth. (page no.94/Farr).

23.abcde---(page no.94/Farr).

24.bcd---In fluoroscopy,automatic brightness control is essential .The area of the output screen used by the ABC system is not full screen.In general ,the brightness in the central area of the screen is selected because the user will have centered the imaging system to the area of radiological interest . (page no.94-

95/Farr).

25.abde----The lower the input dose rate to the intensifier ,the lesser is the noise in the displayed image. (page no.96/Farr).

26.abcde----(page no.97/Farr).

27.bde---- Veiling glare is produced by scattering effects in the image intensifier .It is mainly from light scattering in the output window of the intensifier.Veiling glare is one of causes of central area of the image being brighter than the periphery (vignetting). (page no.98/Farr).

28.bcd----Spatial resolution is tested using a grid test object .Contrast resolution may be tested with a low-contrast test object. (page no.98/Farr).

29.cde---- The image intensifier system has yamma=1 this is in contrast to a film-screen radiography. (page no.93/Farr).

30.bcde---- Change of the voltages of the intermediate electrodes lead to magnification mode of image intensifier .The electron crossover is moved nearer to the input screen. (page no.93/Farr).

31.abcde---(page no.99/Farr).

32.abcde---(page no.101/Farr).

33.abcde---[Page 167/Christensen]

34.abe----Cesium iodide used as input fluorescent is deposited on aluminum substrate by the process of vapor deposition ,which produce needle shaped crystal perpendicular to the aluminum substrate and so there is minimal diffusion of light produced by phosphor layer. [Page 166--167/Christensen]

35.abcde----(page no.100/Farr).

36.abde---In digital substraction

angiography .the substracted image appears more noisier.
----(page no.100-01/Farr).

37.ad----In Dual energy substraction ,the contrast of bone is significantly reduced in high kv.Substracting the low kv image from the high kv image improves soft tissue contrast and minimizes the visualization of bone , and so it is of value in chest radiography.(page no.100 101/Farr).

38.ace-----In pulsed fluoroscopy ,no flickering is seen in static scene at lower pulse rate .The switching is more precise in grid controlled fluoroscopy. (page no.96/Farr).

39.abcde---- ----(page no.95/Farr).

40.ace----Maximum concentration of rods is in the periphery of retin.Rods are most sensitive to ble-green light. (Page 166/Christensen)

41.bcd---Automatic brightness control is essential .The area of the output screen used by the ABC system is not full screen.In general ,the brightness in the central area of the screen is selected because the user will have centered the imaging system to the area of radiological interest . (page no.94-95/Farr).

42.abde----The lower the input dose rate to the intensifier ,the lesser is the noise in the displayed image.
(page no.96/Farr).

CHAPTER 5

Computed Radiography

1.True regarding fourth generation scanner
a.the detectors are arranged in a stationary ring inside the path of the rotating tube
b.overcome some of problems of detector stability and reconstruction made simpler
c.outer part of the fan beam always pass outside the patients
d.during each rotation ,every detector is able to measure attenuated radiation
e.permit the caliberation of each detector throughout the scanning cycle

2.True regarding Compted radiography
a.invented by G.N. Hounsefield,a scientist at EMI Limited in Middlesex,England
b.invention announced in April ,1972
c.invention announced at the Annual Congress of the British Intitute of Radiology
d.mathematical basis established by an Austrian mathematician, J.Radon
e.Oldendorf in 1961 and Cormack in 1963 built lab models of CT

3.True regarding original EMI CT scanner
a.use of water bath to facilitate heat dissipation of CT scan
b.the water bath rotate

independently of head
c.The total number of transmission measurements were 28,800
d.CT image was displayed on 80 x 80 matrix
e.total study time was approximately 25 minutes

4.True regarding CT number
a.represents the average linear attenuation coefficients of tissues within the voxel
b.the value stored in pixel
c.CT number = 1000x (linear attenuation coefficients of tissue – linear attenuation coefficients of water) / linear attenuation coefficients of water
d.term hounsfield unit is used for CT number
e.fat and water are used for the caliberation of the CT number of the scale of the scanner

5.True regarding gas-filled detector
a.different shape and size
b.use of ionization of inert gas by the incoming radiation to produce a signal
c.voltage between the anode and cathode determines the mode of operation
d.an ionization chamber operate at low voltage
e.the current produced is directly proportional to the intensity of the

incoming radiation in all modes

6.True regarding generation of CT scan

a.use of fan-shaped x ray beam in 2nd, 3rd and 4th generation CT scan

b.use of multiple detectors in 2nd, 3rd and 4th generation CT scan

c.shortening of scan time in 2nd, 3rd and 4th generation CT scan

d.only linear type of x ray tube movement in 2st generation CT scan

e.more linear movements of x ray tube in 2nd generation than in 1st generation

7.True regarding 3rd generation CT scanner(fan beam geometry)

a.the General Electric Company introduced 2rd generation CT scan

b.no translatory motion of xray tube

c.both x ray tube and detectors rotate around the patients in concentric circles(rotate-rotate)

d.the detectors and x ray tube are in precise alignment throughout the entire scan motion

e.both xenon and scintillation crystal detectors can be used

8.True regarding 4th generation CT scan

a.the detectors donot move

b.the detectors form a ring that completely surrounds the patients

c.the x ray tube rotates in a circle outside the detector ring

d.there is clear advantage of 4rd and 3th generation over each other

e.some designs have more than 2000 detectors

9.True regarding fan beam/multiple detector array CT scan

a.used in 1st generation CT scan

b.shortening of scan/increased speed great advantage

c.increased scattered radiation is principal disadvantage

d.rotate-rotate and rotate-fixed CT scan cnnot achieve scan times much shorter than 1sec

e.the total number of Compton reaction is more in pencil beam scanner than fan beam scanners

10.True regarding spiral scanning

a.slice width cannot be less than the detector width

b.slice width cannot be multiples of the detector width

c.high scan speed

d.possibility of slice misregistration

e.greater load on x ray tube

11.True regarding detectors in CT scan

a.rotate-fixed scanners (4th generation) must use scintillation crystal detectors

b.xenon gas ionization detectors are limited in use to rotate-rotate type(3rd generation) of scanner

c. rotate-rotate type(3rd generation) of scanner may use scintillation crystal detectors

d.the first two generation of scanners used thallium-activated sodium iodide scintillation crystals and photomultiplier

e.cadmium tungstate is most commonly used scintillation detectors

12.True regarding scintillation crystals

a.produce light on interaction with ionizing radiation

b.normally made of tiny crystals embedded in the matrix

c.polished surfaces to facilitate extraction of the light

d.look alike a piece of clear glass or plexiglass

e.sodium iodide is an example

13.True regarding scintillation crystals

a.emit light photon inversely proportional to the energy of the incident x ray photons

b.afterglow noted in all crystals

c.the color of light depend on type of crystal and its activator (dopant)

d.all crystal must be matched to a light detector

e.thullium activated sodium iodide scintillation crystal used in 1st and 2nd generation scan

14.True regarding scintillation detector

a.NaI is hygroscopic and requires an air- tight container

b.NaI has a very long afterglow ,so not suitable for fast scan

c.photomultiplier tubes are fairly large,so not suitable for current CT geometry

d.photodiodes offer the advantage of smaller size ,greater stability and lower cost

e.90% of light in NaI is emitted over a time of 150ms

15.Example of scintillation crystals is/are

a.NaI

b.Cesium iodide

c.bismuth germinate

d.cadmium tungstate

e.barium sulphate

16.True regarding approximate range of CT numbers for various tissues

a.air   (-1000)

b.water (0)

c.bone (500-1500)

d.muscle (40-60)

e.grey matter of brain (35-45)

17.True regarding scintillation detectors

a.cadmium tungstate doenot have afterglow problem

b.with rotate-fixed geometry ,alignment between rotaing x ray tube and fixed detectors is fixed

c.highly efficient crystal reduces crosstalk

d.detectors with high stopping power promote crosstalk

e.crosstalk reduces resolution

18.True regarding gas filled detector

a.Gieger counter operate at low voltage

b.proportional counter operate at low voltage

c.output signal is proportional to the energy of the photon in proportional counter

d.hand carried survey meters are Geiger counter type of detector

e.xenon gas ionization chamber is used in CT scan

19.True regarding artefact

a.ring artefact appear as a light or dark ring seen in the image

b.ring artefact is due to detector malfunction (giving too low or to high signal)

c.ring artefact is seen in only single slice scanner,not in multi-slice scanner

d.Cone beam artefact leads to blurring at the boundaries between high-contrast details

e.cupping in the image is seen due to partial volume effect

20.True regarding cone beam effect
a.assume x ray beam is non-divergent in the z-direction
b.signinficant in single slice CT scan
c.becomes more significant with increased numbers of slices
d.becomes more significant with increasing detector length
e.cone beam algorithm is used to eccentuate the effect

21.True regarding Scanned projection radiographs
a.also known as scanogram,scout view,topogram
b.a transmission image taken at a fixed projection angle
c.the collimator is generally set to the widest slice width
d.poor spatial resolution better with a standard radiograph
e.used for planning the CT sequence

22.True regarding beam hardening artefact
a.there is hardening of x ray beam as it crosses the patients due to filtering of low energy photons
b.attenuation coefficient and the CT number of a given tissues increase along the beam path
c.CT numbers are lower in the periphery of the patients (inverse cupping)
d.may produce dark streaks in the image
e.may be reduced by beam hardening artefact and bow-tie filter

23.True regarding xenon gas chamber
a.used in CT scan as detectors
b.xenon gas used ,being heaviest among the inert gas (atomic number-54)
c.xenon compressed by 8 to 10 atmoshpheric pressure to increase its density
d.long size of chamber,so not used in rotate-fixed CT scan
e.low efficiency (50 to 60 %) due to low density and absorption of x ray by the front window

24.True regarding x ray attenuation
a.depend on composition of tissue
b.independet of thickness of tissue
c.depend on quality of the x ray beam
d.the linear attenuation coefficient is same for monochromatic and polychromatic beam
e.weighting factor is taken into account to compensate the difference between the size and shape of the scanning beam and the picture matrix

25.True regarding methods of image reconstruction
a.determine the linear attenuation coefficients of all pixels in the image matrix
b.attempt ot solve the linear attenuation coefficients as rapidly as possible without compromising the accuracy
c.The original EMI scanner took 4 to 5 minutes to process the data for a single CT section
d.Back- projection (summation method) is the oldest means of image reconstruction
e.An algorithm is a mathematical method for solving a problem

26.True regarding back-projection
a.it is oldest means of image

construction ,but widely used

b.all points in the back projected image receive density contributions from neighboring structures

c.the height of the steps is proportional to the amount of radiation that passed through the block

d.the steps are assigned to a gray scale density that is proportional to their height and arranged in rows called "rays"

e.rays are superimposed (backprojected) to produce a crude reproduction of the original object

27.True regarding Iterative methods of image reconstruction

a.starts with an assumption

b.comparison of assumption with measured values

c.correction to bring assumption and measured value into disagreement

d.the over and over repeating of process of correction until assumed and measured values are the same or within acceptable limits

e.the correction sequence may involve the whole matrix,one ray ,or a single point(simultaneous reconstruction,ray-by-ray correction,point-by-point correction)

28.True regarding analytic methods of image reconstruction

a.exact formulas used

b.Fourier analysis is based on fact that any function of time or space can be represented by the sum of various frequencies and amplitudes of sine and cosine waves

c.the projected information is filtered in filtered back

projection(frequencies for blurring is filtered)

e.faster than iterative method (secs cs minutes) in incomplete method

e.with insufficient data ,iterative method is superior than analytic method

29.True regarding CT number

a.reflects a relationship between the linear absorption coefficient for a pixel with that of water

b.In currently available CT units,K has a value of 1000

c.CT number allows the computer to present the information as a picture with a large gray scale

d.CT numbers based on a magnification constant of 500 are called Hounsfield units(H)

e.water has linear attenuation coefficients of 0.191/cm

30.True regarding CT number

a.window level refers to the center CT number

b.window width refers to the range of CT numbers above and below the window level

c.window level and window width are set by the operator

d.CT number of water is 0 (zero) and that of air is -1000(minus thousand)

e.windowing limits viewing to a narrow portion of the total information available

31.True regarding Quantum Mottle(noise) in CT scan

a.refers to variation in the number of x ray photons absorbed by the detector

b.the only way to decrease noise is to decrease the number of photons absorbed by the detector c.the way to increase the number of photons absorbed is to increase x ray dose to the patients

d.Contemporary scanners have noise values in the range of 0 1 to to 4 %

e.Pixels must vary by more than 2 to 4HU for the variation to be statistically significant

32. True regarding noise

a.due to the statistical emission of photons from the x ray tube

b.the statistical fluctuation is function of number of photons,increasing with increasing counts

c.the mottle becomes more visible as the accuracy of the reconstruction improves

d.most of noise in current CT images is due to improvement in mathematical reconstruction

e.Counting statistics are intimately related to voxel size.

33. Regarding collimators in CT scan

a.collimated at two points

b.collimator at the detector is sole means of controlling scatter radiation

c.collimator doesnot regulate the thickness of the tomographic slice (the voxel length)

d.collimators determine pixel size

e.coliimator at x ray tube and and that at the detector is perfectly aligned

34. True regarding dosing in the CT scan

a.CT resposnsible for 40% of total population dose that is attributed to medical exposures in UK

b.CT exam is responsible for only 4% of the total dose that use ioninsing radiation

c.multislice scanner delivers somewhat higher dose than single – slice scanners

d.the CT dose index is a measure of dose from single rotation of the gantry

e.CTDI is measured using a pencil ionization chamber

35. True regarding first CT scan generation

a.use of single detector per tomographic section

b.x ray tube detector movement – both linear and rotator

c.use of pencil-like x ray beam

d.original EMI CT scanner belongs to 1st generation

e.scan time of the order of seconds

36. True regarding spatial resolution of CT

a.ability to display separate images of two objects placed close together

b.spatial and contrast resolution are independent of each other

c.contrast and spatial resolution are intimately related to the radiation dose absorbed by the detector

d.attempt to improve spatial resolution may cause increased noise level and decreased contrast level

e.the test objects of high contrast are used for measurement .

37. True regarding spatial resolution in CT

a.detector size place a limit on maximum spatial resolution

b.to record a pair line ,there should be one detector for one line pair. the opaque line and one detector for the space adjacent to the opaque line

c.resolution of 10 line pairs per cm means the same as resolution of 0.5 mm

d.to record a line pair .there should be a minimum of one pixel for an opaque line and one pixel for the adjacent space

e.the reconstruction matrix must be large enough to reconstruct all available information

38. True regarding spatial resolution in CT scan

a.the maximum high-contrast spatial resolution that may be achieved is about 20 lp cm^{-1}

b.high contrast spatial resolution within the scan plane is limited by pixel size

c.pixel size is an intrinsic limitation

d.the alogrithm used affect resolution

e.width of the projection path of X –ray beam affect the spatial resolution

39. True regarding CT dose index (CDTI)

a.Dose- length product $=CTDI_{VOL}$ x the total scan length

b.E/DLP is much lower in head than for the regions in trunk

c.E/DLP is lower for chest than for scans involving the pelvis

d.highest E/DLP is associated with scans of pelvis due to highest W_T foe gonads

e.effective dose of head CT is 1.5 mSv

40. True spatial resolution of CT scan

a.focal spot size ,geometry of scanner,sensitive area of the detector affect spatial resolution

b.spatial resolution increases with sampling frequency

c.no significant difference in spatial resolution in transaxial plane in axial and helical scanning

d.spatial resolution in the z-plane depend on slice thickness

e.spatial resolution depend on pitch

41. True regarding patients dose.

a.in principle ,the number of detector rows has no influence on dose

b.the reconstruction algorithm and FOV has marked influence on patients dose

c.more patients dose with multislice scanner rather than single –slice scanner

d.over-scanning and over-collimation increases patients dose

e.dose is inversely proportional to pitch

42. True regarding computed radiography

a. the commonest means of acquiring plain radiographic images in a digital format

b. Photostimulable phosphor plates replace the conventional film/screen combination in a cassette

c. can be used with standard X-ray equipment and fluoroscopy

d. produce a latent image by promoting electrons to metastable traps of lower energy level

e. plate is 'read out' in raster fashion by a scanning laser beam in the plate reader

43. True regarding CT scan artefact

a. motion artefact is no more seen

b.streak artefact refers to artefact at

the edge of high contrast objects

c.beam hardening effect are minimized by reconstruction programs

d.ring artefact is due to occaisional beakdown of x ray tube

e.motion artefact is primary reason for development of faster scan

44.True regarding artefact

a.reconstruction programme overcome motion artefact

b.an object in motion appear as a steak in the opposite to direction of motion

c.motion of metallic or gas – containing structures produce steak artefact

d.severe reduction of transmission of x ray by high density material produce steak artfefact

e.steak artefact due to violation of assumption that each detector ,at every position ,observe some transmitted radiation.

45.True regarding Beam-Hardening artefact

a.beam hardening is due to absorption of low energy photons from heterochromatic x ray beam

b.there is variation in linear attenuation coefficient due to beam hardening

c.reconstruction programme anticipate and correct the beam hardening effect to very high precision

d.cup artefact in the head is dur to steak effect

e.ring aretefact is due to miscaliberation of one detector in a rotate-rotate geometry scanner

46.True regarding Compted radiography

a.invented by G.N. Hounsefield,a scientist at EMI Limited in Middlesex,England

b.invention announced in April ,1972

c.invention announced at the Annual Congress of the British Intitute of Radiology

d.mathematical basis established by an Austrian mathematician, J.Radon

e.Oldendorf in 1961 and Cormack in 1963 built lab models of CT

47.True regarding computed tomography

a.generates images in transaxial sections

b.CT images not influenced by the properties of neighbouring regions of the body

c.CT was introduced in the early 1970s

d.methods of CT image reconstruction discovered decades before CT scan introduction

e.Computer technology developments has much effect on CT growth.

48.True regarding patients dose

a.radiation output increases by about 40% for an increase of 20 kV

b.there is a direct relationship between mAs and dose

c.use of m A modulation technique may reduce dose in the range of 10-40%

d.in single- slice scanner ,patients dose is generally independent of slice width

e.patients dose is directly proportional to pitch

49.True regarding approximate range of CT numbers of various tissues

a.white matter (20-30)
b.fat (-60 to -150)
c.lung (-300 to -800)
d.air (-1000)
e.bone (500-1500)

50.True regarding photon starvation

a.a variant of the steak artefact
b.typically seen in pelvic scan with bilateral hip implants
c.due to very high x ray attenuation outside the dynamic range of the processing unit
d.tissues between the hips are poorly represented in the displayed image
e.horizontal steaks appear across the image

51.True regarding CT image

a.partial volume effect on the image depends on the thickness of the transaxial image
b.partial volume effect reduce the visibility of high- contrast detail
c.a high contrast object that is smaller than the voxel is not seen due to partial volume effect
d.eye have limited capacity to distinguish levels of gray (about 50)
e.windowing bring about the hidden detail in the image

52.True regarding CT dose index (CDTI)

a.Cylindrical Perspex phantom is used for its measurement
b.$CTDI_w$ is in range of 100-400 mGy for most standard scanning protocols
c.$CTDI_{vol}$ is an approximation to the average absorbed dose within the scanned volume
d.Maximum skin dose is approximately equal to $CTDI_w$ for scans of head and about 20% higher for body scans
e.skin dose in CT scan is much higher than prolonged fluoroscopy

53.True regarding X-ray tubes of CT scanner

a.anode-cathode axis parallel to the axis of rotation of the scanner to minimize heel effect
b.typically have two focal spots ,the smallest being about 0.6mm
c.heat capacities of 4MJ or more
d.incorporation of heat exchanger to cool oil
e.typically scanners are operated at 120 kv

54.True regarding CT scanner

a.rotate-translate type of CT scanner belong to first and second generation scanner
b.time taken by second generation scanner for data acquisition for single slice is less than 20s
c.there is no need for linear translation of tube and detectors in second generation scanner
d.third generation scanner allows for continuous data collection through a full 360 rotation
e.rotate- rotate scanner belong to fourth generation scanner

55.True regarding computed radiography

a. the commonest means of acquiring plain radiographic images in a digital format
b. Photostimulable phosphor plates replace the conventional film/screen combination in a cassette
c. can be used with standard X-ray equipment and fluoroscopy
d. produce a latent image by

promoting electrons to metastable traps of lower energy level

e. plate is 'read out' in raster fashion by a scanning laser beam in the plate reader

56.True regarding CT

a.total number of detectors increased in fourth generation scanner

b.higher dose in fourth generation scanner

c.electron beam scanner is known as fifth-generation scanner

d.electron beam scanner was designed for imaging of the heart

e.third generation geometry has become standard for multislice scanners

57.True regarding post precessing technique in CT scan

a. MPR and curved planar reconstruction (CPR)— allows the image to be viewed in any plane chosen, including a curved plane with CPR

b. MIP displays the highest attenuation voxels in an image only, thus allowing visualization of structures (usually vessels) not in a single plane

c. SSD gives 3D representations of the anatomy in grey scale

d. VR allows visualization of the vessels distinct from the surrounding anatomy (useful in cerebral angiography)

e. SSD is not prone to noise and artefacts.

58.True regarding pixel and voxel

a.matrix size is the number of points in a picture matrix ,6400 (80 x 80)

b.field size refers to the outside dimentions of the CT slice

c.field size dictates the maximum size of an anatomic part that can be examined

d.The scan field of view generally ranges from about 40cm to 50cm

e.resolution is a function of pixel size,same resolution for same size of pixel

59.True regarding patients dose and resolution in CT

a.typical doses range from about 2 cGy(rad) to about 4.0 cGy

b.improvement of both contrast resolution and spatial resolution requires increased patients dose

c.improved spatial resolution requires larger pixel size

d.dose rates have improved in higher generation of CT scan

e.contrast resolution improves only if counting statistics improve

60.True regarding the requirements of CT scanner detectors

a.small size in order to allow good spatial resolution

b.to have high detection efficiency

c.to have fast response with negligible afterglow

d.to have norrow dynamic range

e.to have a stable ,noise-free response

61.True regarding the ionization chamber detectors

a.elongated in the direction parallel to the X-ray beam

b.use of xenon gas because of high atomic number(54) and K-shell binding energy(35keV)

c.pressure of gas about 20atm/2Mpa

d.detection efficiency of 90%

e.highly useful in multislice scanner

62. True regarding solid state detectors used in multislice scanner

a.a scintillant with an embedded silicon photodiode to detect light output

b.cadmium tungstate ,bismuth germinate ,rare earth ceramic are used as scintillant

c.the overall the detection efficiency is close to 80%

d.can be very small down to about 1x0.5 mm^2

e.have negligible afterglow and stable response

63. True regarding bow tie filters

a.thin at centre and progressively thicker towards the edges of the fan beam

b.minimize the unnecessary high dose at the periphery of patients.

c.equalize the transmitted intensities emerging from the patients

d.even out the beam- hardening effect across the projected fan beam

e.it is so called because of shape

64. True regarding image reconstruction

a.alogrithms refers to complex mathematical technique used for reconstruction of CT image

b.most algorithms are based on the method of back-projection

c.filtering is a mathematical process to overcome the blurring of image produced by back projection

d.filtered back projection is the most common method used for image reconstruction

e.there are different filters and back-projection algorithms

65. True regarding Computed tomography fluoroscopy

a.display of CT image in real time

b.continuous rotation of the gantry with table movement

c.most common use for biopsy needle placement

d.risk of relatively high patients skin doses

e.use of fast reconstruction techniques ,generally from 180 degree data sets

66. True regarding slip ring technology

a.permits continuous ,unidirectional rotaion of the x-ray tube and detectors around the patients

b.introduced in early 1980s

c.comprises metal ring mounted on the gantry

d.connected to the signal output from the detectors

e.the connector is able to retain good contact with the ring as the gantry rotates

67. True regarding single –slice volume ,spiral or helical CT

a.faster rotation times

b.continuous acquisition of data

c.Pitch =tabletop movement per rotation/slice thickness x 2

d.no need of interpolation of measured data to reconstruct the image

e.the position of the reconstructed section scan be selected retrospectively as required

68. True regarding CT scan

a.generally scanners have a total tube filtration of about 6 mm aluminium

b.Cupper filter is necessary in CT scan

c.post- patients collimator is meant

to reduce scatter radiation

d.post-patients collimation is neither necessary nor possible for multislice scanners

e.bow tie filters is useless in CT scan

69.True regarding CT dose index (CDTI)

a.measure of dose from a single rotaion of the gantry

b.useful parameter to assess the dose within the scan plane

c.useful for describing the dose efficiency of a scan protocol

d.useful for comparisons between scan model

e. less useful for a comparison of doses to individual patients

70.True regarding CT resolution

a.increasing the matrix size improve high contrast spatial resolution

b.decreasing pixel size decrease high contrast spatial resolution

c.linear attenuation coefficients of water and plexiglass differ by 32% at an effective energy of 70 keV

d.high contrast resolution is pixel – size limited.

e.whole picture element appears white even with small amount of calcium due to partial volume averaging.

71.True regarding contrast resolution

a.it is ability to disply object that is only slightly different in density from its surroundings

b.low contrast visibility is determined by noise

c.homogeneity of background is a function of noise

d.contemporary CT can disply objects 3 mm in diameter with density difference of 0.5 % or less.

e.a density difference of about 10% is required for contrast resolution in fil-screen radiography

72.True regarding pitch

a.pitch above 1 reduce exposure time

b.pitch above 1 reduce patients dose

c.increase in pitch increase resolution and need more interpolation

d.increasing pitch beyond 2 gives unacceptable image

e.pitch is increased beyond 1.5 for most clinical applications

73.True regarding CT imaging

A.true three- dimensional imaging requires isotropy

b.voxel size must unequal in all three dimensions for three dimensional imaging

c.voxel size in the three transaxial plane is determined by the matrix size and the field of view

d.isotropic data can be reconstructed in only transaxial plane

e.maximum intensity projections is used for angiography

74.True regarding pencil dose ionization chamber used for CT dose index measurement

a.typical diameter about 8mm

b.typical length about 100mm

c.width is significantly greater than the maximum slice width

d.measured dose multiplied by the diameter of the chamber represents the integration of dose profile

e.CTDI= dose integrated over the complete dose profile /nominal slice width

75.True regarding the multislice scanner

a.use solid state detectors with multiple rows of detectors
b.the length of the detector along the z-axis determines the reconstructed slice width
c. the width collimated fan beam determines the reconstructed image
d.beam pitch = tabletop movement per rotation/collimator length
e.slice or row = tabletop movement per rotation/slice width

76.True regarding pixel

a.pixel is a picture element
b.pixel is a flat surface without thickness
c.a given size of pixel does not depend on size of appear on size of TV monitor
d.a pixel size represent the different area in patient
e.voxel add adds the third dimention to the area represented by the pixel

77.True regarding computed radiography

a.multiple projections of object is used to reconstruct the internal structure of an object
b.image quality is related to the number of ray projections used to reconstruct each CT scan image
c.each ray is assumed to contain new information (non-redundant information)
d.the original EMI scanner was designed specifically for evaluation of the brain
e.The detector used in original EMI scanner were sodium iodide scintillation crystals coupled to photomultiplier tubes

78.True regarding original EMI CT scanner

a.use of oil-cooled rotating anode
b.Nominal focal spot size ---2.25 x 12mm
c.tube operating parameters---120 kVp and 33 m A
d.poorly filtered with a half-value layer of 6 mm of aluminium(0.22mm of cupper)
e.use of a pair of detector and another reference detectors

79.True regarding image processing

a.three-dimensional surface rendering is achieved by selecting suitable range of CT numbers
b.maximum intensity projection is used for CT angiography
c. minimum intensity projection is used for imaging the tracheobronchial region
d.varying level of opacity and different colors are used in three-dimensional volume-rendering
e.vertual endoscopy is used to display the internal walls of body structures such as the colon

80.True regarding quantum noise in CT scan

a.S/N ratio is directly related to the square root of the number of photons detected
b.S/N is incearsed by the square root of m A s
c.S/N is decreased by the square root of slice width
d.increased field of view and matrix size reduces noise
e.increasing Kv reduce noise

81.True regarding noise in CT scan

a.pitch does not affect the noise in single-slice scanners
b.noise increases with pitch in

multislice scanners

c.noise become more apparent as window width is reduced

d.electronic noise is least significant among other kind of noise

e.quantum noise is reduced by increasing Kv

82.True regarding streak artefact

a.appear as black and white band

b.produced by cardiac motion

c.produced by mechanical misalignment and movements of the patients

c.produced by high attenuation objects (metal implants ,dental amalgam)

d.small areas of bone or contrast medium may produce streak artefacts

e.metal correction algorithms may accentuate steak artefact

Answer
Computed Radiography

1.bce---In fourth generation scanner the detectors are arranged in a stationary ring outside the path of the rotating tube.During each rotation ,every detector is able to measure unattenuated radiation which permit the caliberation of each detector throughout the scanning cycle. (page no.106/Farr).

2.abcde----[Page 237-40/Christensen].

3.bcde---In original EMI CT scanner ,the patients head was incorporated into water bath to facilitate data analysis within the computer. A slip ring between the rubber head cap and water bath allowed the bath to rotate independently of the head.[Page 291-293/Christensen].

4.abcd----Air and water are used for the caliberation of the CT number of the scale of the scanner (page no.104/Farr).

5.abcd--- Current produced is directly proportional to the intensity of the incoming radiation at low voltage (ionization chamber) .[Page 299/Christensen].

6.abc---X-ray tube movement is both rotator and linear in 2st generation CT scan but there is less linear movements of x ray tube in 2nd generation than in 1st generation .[Page 299/Christensen].

7.abcde----.[Page 294 95/Christensen].

8.abe--- The x ray tube rotates in a circle inside the detector ring in the 4th generation CT scan.There is no clear advantage of 4rd and 3th generation over each other. .[Page 295-296/Christensen].

9.bcd---- Fan beam/multiple detector array is not used in 1st generation CT scan.The total number of Compton reaction is nearly samefor pencil beam and fan beam scanners,but tha scattered photons are more likely to be recorded by the fan beam unit. .[Page 296/Christensen].

10.ace—In spiral scanning ,slice width can be multiples of the detector width and thnere is no possibility of slice misregistration .[Page 111/Christensen].

11.abcde---[Page 298/Christensen].

12.acde----[Page 298/Christensen]. Scintillation crystal is normally made of single crystal of material.

13.cde--- Scintillation crystals emit light photon directly proportional to the energy of the incident x ray photons. Light photons emitted with delay (afterglow) is noted in some type of crystals [Page 298/Christensen].

14.abcd---9% of light in NaI is emitted over a time of 150ms. [Page 298/Christensen].

15.abcd-----[Page 298/Christensen].

16.abcde-----(page no.104/Farr).

17.ace--- With rotate-fixed geometry ,alignment between rotaing x ray tube and fixed detectors is constantly changing because the geometry dictates that the detectors must be aligned with the center of rotation and the x ray tube. Detectors with high stopping power reduce crosstalk. [Page 299/Christensen].

18.cde---Gieger counter operate at high voltage,proportional counter operate at intermediate voltage while ionization chamber operate at low voltage.Secondary electrons are produced in proportional and Geiger counter.(Page 300 / Christensen].

19.abd-----Ring artefact is seen both single slice scanner and in multi-slice scanner .Cupping in the image is seen due to beam hardening artefact. -----(page no.116/Farr).

20.cd---Standard reconstruction algorithm assume that x ray beam is non-divergent in the z-direction and it is not signinficant in single slice CT scan.Cone beam algorithm is used to minimize the significance of this effect. -----(page no.113/Farr).

21.abe----In Scanned projection radiographs , the collimator is generally set to the narrowest slice width and spatial resolution is compared with a standard radiograph . (page no.109-10/Farr).

22.ade-----Due to beam hardening artefact ,attenuation coefficient and the CT number of a given tissues decrease along the beam path and so CT numbers are lower in the centre of the patients (cupping). (page no.115/Farr).

23.abcde----.(Page 300 / Christensen].

24.abce----The xray attenuation is not independent of tissue thickness.The linear attenuation coefficient is not same for monochromatic and polychromatic beam.The linear attenuation coefficient of a heterochromatic beam decreases as filtration increases its mean energy. -.(Page 301-303 / Christensen].

25.abcde-----(Page 303-304 / Christensen].

26.bcde--- It is oldest means of image construction ,but not widely used. .(Page 303-304 / Christensen].

27.abde--- Iterative methods of image reconstruction starts with an assumption which is compared with measured values. Correction is done to bring assumption and measured value into agreement. .(Page 306 / Christensen].

28.abce------Analytic method is faster than iterative method (secs cs minutes in complete data.With insufficient data ,iterative method is superior than analytic method .for complete data both methods are equally accurate. .(Page 307 / Christensen].

29.abde----- CT number reflects a relationship between the linear absorption coefficient for a pixel with that of water.CT number =K(magnification constant) x pixel linear attenuation constant –water linear attenuation constant/ water

linear attenuation constant.CT numbers based on a magnification constant of 1000 are called Hounsfield units(H) in honor of Hounsfield.
.(Page 308 / Christensen].

30.abcde---.(Page 309 / Christensen].

31.ace-----In CT scan Only way to decrease noise is to increase the number of photons absorbed by the detector.Contemporary scanners have noise values in the range of 0.2 to 0.4 %.
.(Page 310 / Christensen].

32.ace--- Noise is due to the statistical emission of photons from the x ray tube,and the statistical fluctuation is function of number of photons decreasing with increasing counts.Most of noise in current CT images is result of statistical fluctuations and is not related to the mathematical reconstruction.
.(Page 310-12 / Christensen].

33.abe---Collimator regulate the thickness of the tomographic slice (the voxel length).collimators does not determine pixel size.The pixel size is determined by the computer program. .(Page 296 / Christensen].

34.abcde----(Page 116 / Christensen].

35.abcd--- First CT scan generations can takes approx ,25minutes for five-view study of the head. .(Page 293 / Christensen].

36.acd---Spatial and contrast resolution are intimately related to each other . The test objects of high contrast are used for measurement (Page 314 / Christensen].

37.acde---- Detector size place a limit on maximum spatial resolution in CT scan .To record a pair line ,there should be one detector for the opaque line and one detector for the space adjacent to the opaque line.
.(Page 314-15 / Christensen].

38.abde----- Spatial resolution in CT scan,high contrast spatial resolution within the scan plane is limited by pixel size which is not an intrinsic limitation because it depend on matrix size and FOV.
.(Page 114 / Christensen].

39.abcde----(page no.117/Farr).
40.abcde--- ----(pageno.114/Farr).
41.abcde--- ----(pageno.117/Farr).
42.abe-----Computed radiography can be used with standard X-ray equipment but not for fluoroscopy. It produce a latent image by promoting electrons to metastable traps of higher energy level(CHAPTER 1 ,Adam: Grainger)

43.bce---- Motion artefact has diminished but not eliminated.Ring artefact is due failure of a detector.(Page 318/ Christensen].

44.cde---Reconstruction programme has no ability to make appropriate corrections because motion is random and unprectable .An object in motion appear as a steak in the direction of motion. (Page 318-19 / Christensen].

45.abde--- Reconstruction programme anticipate beam-Hardening artefact and correction of the beam hardening effect is not precise. .(Page 320 / Christensen].

46.abcde.---(Page 237-40/ Christensen].

47.abcde-----.(Page 103-4 / Farr].

48.abcd---Patients dose is inversely proportional to pitch and therefore the use of a pitch of 1.5 rather than 1 leads to a 33% dose rduction. (Page 117 / Farr].

49.abcde----.(Page 115 / Farr].

50.abcde----.(Page 104 / Farr].

51.ade----Partial volume effect reduce the visibility of low- contrast detail.A high contrast object that is smaller than the voxel is seen due to partial volume effect. (Page 104-5 / Farr].

52.acd----$CTDI_w$ is in range of 10-40 mGy for most standard scanning protocols. Skin dose in CT scan is much higher than for radiographic examinations but not as high as doses from prolonged fluoroscopy. (Page 117 / Farr].

53.bcde--- In X-ray tubes of CT scanner, anode-cathode axis remains parallel to the axis of rotation of the scanner to minimize heel effect. (Page 104-5 / Farr].

54.abd----There is need for linear translation of tube and detectors in first and second generation scanner.Rotate- rotate scanner belong to third generation scanner. (Page 104-5 / Farr].

55.abe-----Computed radiography can be used with standard X-ray equipment but not for fluoroscopy. It produce a latent image by promoting electrons to metastable traps of higher energy level(Chapter 1 ,Adam: Grainger)

56.abcde-----(Page 104-5 / Farr].

57.abcd----- SSD gives 3D representations of the anatomy in grey scale, but is prone to noise and artefacts. (Chapter 4 ,Adam: Grainger)

58.abcde-----(Page 312-13Christensen].

59.abe----Improved spatial resolution requires smaller pixel size.Dose rates have remained the same in all types of CT scanners. (Page 318 / Farr].

60.abce ----CT scanner detectors should have to have fast response with negligible afterglow and have wide dynamic range.(Page 107/ Farr].

61.abc--- The ionization chamber detectors has detection efficiency of 60% and are not useful in multislice scanner. ----.(Page 108 / Farr].

62.abcde----.(Page 108 / Farr].

63.abcde----.(Page 107 / Farr].

64.abcde----.(Page 108 / Farr].

65.acde-In Computed tomography fluoroscopy,there is continuous rotation of the gantry without table movement. (Page 110 / Farr].

66.abcde ----.(Page 110 / Farr].

67.abe----In volume ,spiral or helical CT, Pitch =tabletop movement per rotation/slice thickness and measured data need to be interpolated to reconstruct the image. (Page 111 / Farr].

68.acd----In CT scan, Cupper filter is not necessary in CT scan because of improvements in reconstruction algorithms.Bow tie filters is useful in CT scan. (Page 107/ Farr].

69.abcde----.(Page 116-17 / Farr].

70.ade----Decreasing pixel size decreases high contrast spatial resolution.Linear attenuation coefficients of water and plexiglass differ by 12% at an effective energy of 70 keV. (Page 316 / Farr].

71.abcde----.(Page 316-17 / Farr].

72.abd----Increase in pitch reduce resolution because of more interpolation.Pitch is not increased beyond 1.5 for most clinical applications.(Page 111 / Farr].

73.ace----True three- dimensional imaging requires isotropy.Voxel size must be equal in all three dimensions for three dimensional imaging.isotropic data can be reconstructed on any plane.(Page 111 / Farr].

74.abe----Pencil dose ionization chamber used for CT dose index measurement has typical diameter of about 8mm and typical length of about 100mm ,so length is significantly greater than the maximum slice width.Measured dose multiplied by the length of the chamber represents the integration of dose profile .(Page 116-17 / Farr].

75.abde----In the multislice scanner, the width collimated fan beam doesnot determines the reconstructed image. (Page 112/ Farr].

76.abe----A size of pixel depend on size of TV monitor,appear larger on larger monitor.A pixel size represent the same area in patient . (Page 312/ Farr].

77.abcde----.(Page 291-293 / Farr].

78.bce---Original EMI CT scanner uses of oil-cooled stationary anode and was heavily filtered with a half-value layer of 6 mm of aluminium (0.22mm of cupper).
[Page 293/Christensen].

79.abcde----.(Page 114 / Farr].

80.abe---- S/N is increased by the square root of slice width,so increasing the slice width reduce noise . Reduced field of view and larger matrix size increases noise as there is smaller detector area defining each pixel. (Page 114 / Farr].

81.abcde----(Page 115 / Farr].

82.abcd-----Metal correction algorithms may minimize steak artefact produced by high attenuation objects.(Page 115/ Farr].

CHAPTER 6

Radiation protection,Dosimetry,Uk Regulations

1.True regarding measurement of X- rays and gamma rays
a.easy to measure absorbed dose in liquid and solids directly
b.absorbed dose of 1Gy cause temperature rise of tissue of not much greater than 10^{-4} degree Celsius (0.1mK)
c.absorbed dose measurement by temperature rise is highly practical
d.conversion factor for muscle is 1.0 to 1.1 over the whole kv range
e.conversion factor for bone is 5 to 1.2 over whole kv range

2.True regarding absorbed dose
a.refers to the energy deposited per unit mass of the stated material
b.the unit of absorbed dose is rad
c.absorbed dose rate is measured in gray /second
d.1 gray =100 rad
e. Unit of absorbed dose in SI unit is gray

3.True regarding Kerma and absorbed dose
a.an acronym for kinetic energy released to matter
b.Kerma refers to the energy transferred per unit mass of irradiated material ,from photons to electrons at the specified position
c.absorbed dose is the energy deposited as ionization and and excitation by secondary electrons at that position
d.for diagnostic purposes .kerma and absorbed dose are equal

e.Kerma applies to x rays ,gamma rays only

4.True regarding ionization chamber
a.fixed shape of chamber
b.chamber wall made of plastic material
c. c.chamber wall lined with graphite
d.chamber volume of 10-30cm^3 suitable for the measurement of scatter radiation
e.thinner wall of chamber for mammography

5.Reasons for using air as the standard material for dosimetry is/are
a.an effective atomic number (7.6) close to that of tissue(7.4)
b.applicable for measurement over a wide range of x rays energies
c.doses (large and small) and dose rates(large and small) are easily and accurately measured
d.universally available with an invariable composition
e. applicable for measurement over a wide range gamma rays energies

6.True regarding thimble chamber
a.the ionization current is measured by a device known as an voltameter
b.the ionization current is inversely proportional to air kerma rate and the total charge collected to air kerma
c.correction for ambient temperature or pressure is large and

duly corrected

d.the sensitivity of an ionization chamber is proportional to volume

e.air is used as standard material for dosimetry

7.True regarding chamber wall of thimble chamber.(Chapter 1,page no.18,second edition (2008),Farr's Physics for Medical Imaging).

a.must be made of air-equivalent material that matches air in terms of its effective atomic number

b.plastic material is used as wall because its effective atomic number is 26

c.silver is deposited on inner wall to make it electrically conducting

d.wall thickness of 0.2mm is sufficient for photoelectrons from 140 kev

d.thicker wall chamber is used for mammography

8.True regarding Dose area product meters

a.meant for assessment of patients dose,mounted on the collimator of x ray tube

b.use of cylinder type ionization chamber

c.area bigger than the maximum beam size at postion of mounting

d.sealed chamber to avoid changes in calibration caused by changes in temperature and pressure

e.the amount of ionization produced is proportional to dose only

9.True regarding radiation

a.intensity is greater for a constant potential than a pulsating potential

b.intensity is greater for lower rather than higher atomic number targets

c.quality is described in terms of the penetrating power of a x ray beam

d.the most complete description of quality is the average/effective energy of the spectrum

e.the greater is the HVL ,the lesser the effective energy

10.True regarding luminescence

a.absorbs energy from an external source

b.re-emits the absorbed energy in the form of visible light

c.in photoluminescence ,external source of energy is radiation

d.there is delayed light emission (delay time of order of 10^{-6} s) in fluorescence

e.phosphor refers to a material that has luminescent properties

11.True regarding luminescence

a.thermoluminescence—light is emitted only following heating of the irradiated material

b.photostimulable luminescence—light is emitted when the irradiated phosphor is exposed to light

c.thermoluminescent dosimetry and optically stimulated luminescence are used for measurement of radiation dose

d.computed radiography is based on process of photostimulable phosphor

e.the intensity of light emitted from a phosphor is proportional to the energy absorbed from the xray or gamma beam

12.correct matching of dosimeter

a.ionisation chamber---dose are product meters

b.lithium fluoride ---personal and patient dosimetry

c.the photographic effect in silver bromide –film badge

d.photoconductivity in silicon diodes –direct reading electronic personal dosimeters

e. photoconductivity in silicon diodes –dosimeters used in quality assurance

13.True regarding intensity or air kerma rate

a. intensity or air kerma rate is approximately proportional to the square of the kv

b. intensity or air kerma rate is proportional to m A

c .intensity or air kerma rate is inversely proportional to the square of the distance F from a point source

d.the energy fluence or air kerma is proportional to the exposure time

e.intensity is decreased as filtration is increased

14.True regarding band in an atom

a.valence band is the outermost band that is completely filled with electrons

b.conduction band remains partially occupied with no electrons

c.forbidden zone describes the energy levels that cannot be occupied by an electron in that material

d.energy band of valence band>forbidden band>conduction band

e.impurities introduce electrons traps (discrete energy shell) in the forbidden zone

15.True regarding luminescence

a.impurities in phosphor is a big problem

b.energy levels of impurities and that of the phosphor is different

c.impurities introduce discrete energy shells within the forbidden zone of phosphor(electron traps)

d.excitation raises electrons from the conduction band into the valence band

e.electrons in the valence band move freely within the material

16.True regarding process of luminescence

a.electrons in conduction band may move in electron trap when such electron come in vicinity of an impure atom

b.when a hole is created in the vicinity of the electron trap, the electron will then fall back into the valence band,generally via the conduction band

c.the holes are created in valence band when the material is irradiated

d.holes are able to travel in valence band

d.light is liberated when trapped electrons fall back to conduction band

17.True regarding radiation damage

a.caused by radiation absorption

b.chemical changes produced within minutes

c.molecular damage occurs immediately

d.biological damage evident in minutes

e.molecular damage follows the chemical changes

18.True regarding luminescence

a.impurities in phosphor is a big problem

b.energy levels of impurities and

that of the phosphor is different
c.impurities introduce discrete energy shells within the forbidden zone of phosphor(electron traps)
d.excitation raises electrons from the conduction band into the valence band
e.electrons in the valence band move freely within the material

19.True regarding process of luminescence

a.electrons in conduction band may move in electron trap when such electron come in vicinity of an impure atom
b.when a hole is created in the vicinity of the electron trap, the electron will then fall back into the valence band,generally via the conduction band
c.the holes are created in valence band when the material is irradiated
d.holes are able to travel in valence band
d.light is liberated when trapped electrons fall back to conduction band

20.True regarding interaction of beta particle with the tissue

a.beta particle in tissue follow a straight path
b.beta particle undergo progressive attenation
c.beta partcicles are easily deflected by orbital electrons
d.total range involved in tissue interaction is of the order of a few centimeters
e.easily absorbed by a few mm of Perspex or by thin sheet of metal

21.True regarding electronic personal dosimeter

a.use simple photodiodes and microelectronics
b.energy resp[onse as good as TLD and film
c.capable of measuring doses im microsievert range (lower than film badge and TLD)
d.can record dose rate and activate in-built alarms
e.no fading of record and can be worn for an indefinite period of time

22.True regarding radiation

a.pure water on irradiation produces a free electron and a positively charged water ion
b.positively charged water ion decomposes immediately and produce hydroxyl free radical and positively charged hydrogen
c.the hydroxyl free radical is highly reactive and powerful reducing agent
d.enzyme damage occurs at molecular level
e.damage at cellular level involves cell death,and cellular transformation

23.True regarding personal dosimeter

a.range of response (film badge— 0.2mGy to 6 Gy ,TLD---0.1mGy to 10^4 Gy
b.linearity of response is noted in film badge,not in TLD
c.maximum time of use (film badge -2 months ,TLD ---12 months)
d.TLD response is dependent on energy
e.film badge is sensitive to temperature and humidity

24.True regarding radiation

a.linear energy transfer (LET) is the sum of the energy deposited in

tissue per unit path length
b.for the same initial energy as an electron ,an alpha particle travels a much shorter distance
c.electron is a high-LET radiation than that of alpha particle
d.damage caused by high-LET radiation is more likely to be repairable
e.relative biological effectiveness explains the difference in radiation effects of different radiation types

25.Correct matching for threshold doses(absorbed dose-Gy) for deterministic effect
a.skin erythema ---2 to 5
b.irreversible skin damage ---20 to 40
c.hair losss---2 to 5
d.sterility ---2 to 3
e.lethality (whole body) –3 to 5

26.True regarding deterministic effect
a.threshold for cataract –5Gy
b.damage to eye is non- cumulative
c.damage to eye has repair mechanism
d.deterministic threshold dose for fetal abnormality ---0.1 to 0.5 Gy
e.fetal exposure may cause spontaneous abortion,birth defect and Down 's syndrome

27.True regarding deterministic effect (non-stochastic effect)
a.no effect below threshold dose
b.the rate at which the dose is delivered influences the threshold dose
c.most deterministic effect have no repair mechanisms
d.greatest fetal abnormality in the third week to third month week of pregnancy

e.large variation in threshold from individual to individual

28.True regarding absorbed dose
a.S.I. unit is Gray in honor of Harold Gray (who developed the Bragg Gray theory)
b.one cGy is the same as one rad (1 gray =100 rad)
c.absorbed dose is dependent of the composition of the radiated material and energy of the beam
d.as a general rule ,the absorbed dose proportional to the degree of attenuation
e.rem is unit of absorbed dose

29.True regading radiosensitivity
a.the more rapidly a cell is dividing ,greater is its sensitivity
b.the lower the degree of functional and morphological,the higher the radiosensitivity
c.spermatogonia,heamatopoetic stem cells,intestinal crypt cells and lymphoma cells are ver radiosensitive
d.differentiated cells are generally relatively radioresistant
e.small lymphocytes ,primary oocytes and neuroblasts are readiosensitive

30.True regarding absorbed dose equivalent
a.measure of biological effectiveness of irradiation
b.rem and sievert (s.i.unit)are units of absorbed dose equivalent
c.one sievert =100 rem
d.rads=rem x quality factor
e.quality factor for x rays is 5

31.True regarding stochastic effect
a.effect arise by chance
b.no threshold dose

c.the risk increases linearly with dose

d.severity of effect does not increases with dose

e.all or none effect

32.True regarding carcinogenesis and organ risk

a.life time study of survivors of Hiroshima and Nagasaki is most significant study of stochastic effects of radiation

b.risk factor for the thyroid cancer is relatively high

c.Overall ,for a uniform whole body irradiation,the risk of fatal cancer is 15% per Sv

d.peak incidence of leukaemias occurs about 7-8yrs after irradiation of red bone marrow

e.latency period for solid tumours os about 40 yrs

33.True regarding fetal irradiation

a.irradiation in utero increase the risk of childhood cancer

b.the risk of developing fatal childhood cancer is 3% per Gy or 1 in 33000 per mGy

c.natural incidence of fatal childhood cancer is 1 in 800

d.a effective dose of 17 mGy is required to double the natural risk of childhood cancer

e.a CT scan of pelvis during pregnancy will quadruple the risk of fatal childhood cancer

34.True regarding stochastic effect of radiation exposure

a.probability of occurrence increases with increasing absorbed dose

b.the severity of the effect depend on the magnitude of the

absorbed dose

c.an-all-none phonenomenon

d. there is a dose threshold

e.examples –cancers and genetic effects

35.Approximate dose to fetus from radiological examination

a.chest PA ---- < 0.01 mGy

b.abdomen or pelvis AP ---1 mGy

c.lumber spine (AP and lateral0---1.5 mGy

d.barium follow through ----2 mGy

e.barium enema ---8 mGy

36.True regarding stochastic effect

a.risk of carcinogenesis is more in younger population

b.no any excess of genetic disorders in the descendants of survivors of Hiroshima and Nagasaki

c.the frequency of congenital defects ,fecundity life expectancy appear to be no different than for the children of nonirradiated parents

d.the average risk over the whole population of hereditary ill health in subsequent children and future generations is estimated to be 1 in 70000 for an exposure of 1mGy to the gonads,

e. the average risk over the reproductive population of hereditary ill health in subsequent children and future generations is estimated to be 1 in 40 000 for an exposure of 1mGy to the gonads,

37.True regarding effective dose

a.the sum value of the weighted organ dose is the effective dose

b.the weighted organ dose =the average equivalent dose to each organ and tissue x tissue weighting factor

c.tissue weighting factor assigned to gonad is 0.01

d.a value of 0.12,0.05 and 0.01 is assigned reapectively to high,moderate and low risk of carcinogenesis

e.the sum of weighting factors is 100

38.True regarding dose area product

a.the product of dose and beam area in units of Gy cm^2 or submultiples

b.cannot be easily measured

c.not related to risk other than that ,for the same examination

d.can be converted to effective dose using conversion factor

e conversion factor used is fixed

39. Approximate dose to fetus from radiological examination

a.CT chest --- 0.1 mGy

b.CT pelvis ---25 mGy

c.T_c-99$_m$ bone scan--- 4 mGy

d. T_c-99$_m$ thyroid scan --- 0.5 mGy

e. T_c-99$_m$ lung perfusion scan --- 0.3 mGy

40.True regarding protection barrier

a.secondary barrier is required for areas protected by a primary barrier

b.use factor (U) for stray radiation is always one (1)

c.correction factor for secondary protection =actual field size/400 (control field size)^2

d.0.2m R is the maximum permissible exposure that the film should receive during its entire storage life

e.the energy of secondary radiation is assumed to be less than to that of the primary radiation

41.True regarding biologic effects of radiation

a.all ionizing radiation are not harmful

b.leukaemia is the most common neoplasia caused by radiation

c.latent period for leukaemia range from 10 to 30 yrs and from 5 to 200 yrs for other tumours

d.the genetic effects of radiation is more frightening than the somatic ones

e.Genetically significant dose is defined as the dose that ,if received by every member of the population,would be expected to produce the same total energy as the actual doses received by various individuals

42.True regarding optical simulated luminescent dosimeters

a.use of aluminium oxide as phosphor

b.emits light in proportion to the dose when exposed to light

c.light source in the reader is laser

d.increased sensitivity down to 0.01 mSv

e.possibility of second reading

43.True regarding electronic dosimeters

a.indirect reading device

b.generally based on Geiger-Muller tubes or silicon diode detectors

c.response energy independent

d.high sensitivity ,able to measure to the nearest 1 microSv

e.expensive

44.True regarding thermoluminescent dosimeters (TLD)

a.used to measure deep and shallow

dose

b. energy dependent response

c.overall sensitivity significantly better than film

d.much less susceptible to environmental effects

e.relatively inexpensive

45.True regarding prerequisite property of radiation used for radiation measurement

a.measurement t should be accurate and unequivocal

b.must be sensitive to producing a large response for a small amount of radiation energy

c.can be converted into absorbed dose

d.measurement independent of intensity

e.must apply equally well to very large and very small doses

46.True regarding terrestrial gamma rays

a.emitted from radioactive materials in the earth crust

b.average exposure due to terrestrial gamma rays is 350microSv/year

c.amount depend on where one live

d.amount depend on the materials used in the construction of the building

e.contribute to 14% of UK population radiation exposure

47.True regarding sources of radiation

a.internal soureces of radiation contribute to radiation exposure of 270 microSv/year

b.potassium-40 contributes about 60% of internal radiation

c. internal soureces of radiation contribute to 14% of UK population radiation exposure

c. Radon contribute to 49% of UK population radiation exposure

c. medical radiation contribute to 14% of UK population radiation exposure

48.True regarding cosmic radiation

a.generated in space such as sun

b.made purely of a broad spectrum of X- and gamma rays

c.mostly attenuated by the atmoshphere

d.the amount is about 320 microSv/year at the sea level

e.the cosmic radiation decreases with altitude

49.True regarding Radon

a.radioactive in nature

b.decay is associated with beta particles

c.produced in the decay chain of uranium

d.highly active gas

e.may permeate through the ground and into the building

50.True regarding factors considered for justification of use of radiation

a.the benefit should exceed the risk to those who are liable to be exposed

b.risk vs dose(risk is proportional to dose)

c.risk vs age (risk is significantly greater for children than for adult)

d.pregnancy and consequent risk to fetus

e. seriousness of illness and resulting outcome from accurate diagnosis

51.True regarding the Health and Safety at Work Act (1974)

a.the act established an advisory

body ,the Health and Safety Commission(HSC) ,and the Health and Safety Executive (HSE)

b.regulations part of the civil law

c.HSE does the policing of compliance with the law

d.HSC has power of inspection and prosecution

e.Uk legislation on health and safety is determined by European directives

52.True regarding radiation exposure in UK

a.Radon represents the largest source of radiation(49%)

b.radon account for radiation exposure of 1.3mSv/year

c.the average dose of radiation is 2.2mSv/year

d.artificial sources of radiation account for an average of 0.4mSv

e.the largest artificial source of radiation is medical radiation

53.True regarding radiation

a.relative biological effectiveness is the ratio of absorbed dose required to induce the same biological end point for two radiation types

b.equivalent dose = absorbed dose x radiation weighting factor

c.Si unit of equivalent dose is sievert (Sv)

d.unit of effective dose is sievert (Sv)

e.effective dose incorporates factors to account for the variable radiosensitivities of organs and tissues in the body

54.True regarding radiation exposures

a.ionisation produces majority of immediate chemical changes in tissue

b.critical molecules for radiation damage are proteins(such as enzymes) and nucleic acids(principally DNA)

c.direct radiation damage is due to rupture of nuclear bonds in the solute molecules

d.indirect radiation damage is due to interaction of solute molecules with free radicles

e.direc radiation damage is more comman than indirect radiation damage

55.correct matching of amount of artificial sources of radiation

a.nuclear weapon tests –4micoSv

b.smoke detectors ---0.1micoSv

c.nuclear discharges—0.3microSv

d.occuptional exposure –6microSv

e.medical radiation ---370microSv

56.True regarding UK legislation

a.HSC have published the three documents—IRR99,ACOP,and Guidance for good pactice

b.IRR 99 concerns the safety of staff and public ,apply to all workplace use of ionising radiations

c.An approved code of practice (ACOP) outlines means of compliance with IRR99

d.Guidance for good pactice has higher status than the ACOP

e.The IRR99 is concerned with the radiation protection of patients

57.True regarding a radiation protection adviser(RPA)

a.may be an employee of the organization or an external consultant

b.The RPA must satisfy the HSE's rquirements for competence

c.in the health service ,the RPA is

almost invariably a radiologist

d.the radiation employer is required to consult a RPA on compliance with the regulations

e.RPA carries out prior risk assessment

58.True regarding radiation protection

a.annual effective dose limit for the lens of the eye for employees and public are 150 mSv and 15 mSv respectively

b.the threshold dose for cataracts is approximately 5 Sv

c.a person at work who received a dose at or close to the dose limit would exceed the dose threshold for cataract after about 35yrs

d. annual effective dose limit for abdomen of emplyess with reproductive capacity is 13 mSv in any consecutive 3-month period .

e. annual effective dose limit for fetus of pregnant employee is 1 mSv over declared term of pregnancy

59.True regarding room design

a.lead (1-2 mm thick) provide sufficient shielding

b.brick or concrete wall (approx 120mm)provide protection equivalent to 1mm of lead

c.calcium plaster is one of the protective material

d.screen panels incorporate 2mm of lead

e.viewing window has no lead to maintain the transparency

60.True regarding radiation sources in the room

a.in fluoroscopy the primary beam is no greater than the size of image receptor

b.the transmitted radiation at the exit side of the patients is no greater than 2% of the primary

c.leakage radition is generally less than 2% of the dose due to scatter

d.scatter is proportional to DAP for a particular radiation geometry

e.scatter radiation is produced within the patients

61.True regarding radiation protection

a.better to have the X- ray tube below the patients

b.overcouch screening table are suitable for interventional studies

c.use of lead apron (0.35mm for general work and 0.5mm for interventional procedures)

d.Barium and tin is incorporated in lead apron to decrease the weight of apron at the cost of efficacy.

e.use of seprate thyroid collar ,and lead glasses or goggles

62.True regading film badge

a.the film badge holder contains a cadmium filter

b.possible to calculate dose for low energy photons and electrons

c.cadmium filter capture alpha particle

d.permanent visual record

e.gives indication of type of radiation

63.True regarding dose limits of pregnant staff

a.dose limit equal to the limit for a member of the public

b.the limit applies over the declared term of pregnancy

c.fetal dose is equal to the dose monitoring reading in diagnostic X-rays imaging

d.restrict the average dose to the abdomen to 13mSv over any consecutive 3-month period

e. .fetal dose is equal 50% of the dose monitoring reading in radionuclide imaging X-rays imaging

64.True regarding ionization chamber and Geiger-Muller counters

a.both respond to x-ray and gamma rays and to fast beta particles

b.the GM tube is less sensitive than the ionization chamber

c.the GM tube is a radiation monitor

d.the GM tube is more compact

e.the GM tube may be used to detect low levels of contamination

65.True regarding IRR99

a.dose limit is relaxed for comforters and carers

b.the employer is required to set dose constraints for comforters and carers

c.dose relaxation can be applied to employees

d.a parent holding young child for x ray position is comforters and carers

e.comforter and carers are kept in dark involved when acting as comforters and carers

66.True regarding radiation protection

a.the effective dose limit is concerned with deterministic risk

b.equivalent dose limits is designed to keep the dose below the thresholds for deterministic effects

c.the dose limits for employees(16-18yrs) is one-tenths of that set for employees above 18yrs or above.

d.the effective annual dose limit for employees and public are 20 mSv and 1mSv respectively

e.the equivalent annual dose limit for skin ,forearm.feet and ankles for employees and public are 500 mSv and 50mSv respectively

67.True regarding controlled area

a.special working procedures needed to restrict radiation exposure

b.likely exposure greater than four-tenths of any dose limit

c.the external dose rate could exceed 7.5microSv/h averaged over the working day

d.x ray room or the injection room used for radionuclide imaging

e.restricted access

68.True regarding contolled area

a.warning signs regarding nature of source (X-rays,radioactive material)

b.warning signs regarding the risk (external radiation,and contamination)

c.area within 4m of X-ray tube and patients for mobile X-ray

d.control on access by the person operating the x ray set

e.person bearing lead apron can be in controlled area during mobile x ray

69.True regarding local rules

a.related to safe methods of working with ionising radiations

b.oral instructions

c.for those working in controlled area only

d.contingency plan

e.describe of controlled and supervised areas

70.True regarding dosimetry

a.the dosimeter services measure the personal dose equivalent

b.the personal dose equivalent at a depth of 20mm is reffered as the deep dose c,deep dose is taken as measure of effective dose

d.shallow dose is taken as measure of the skin dose

e.the standard body badge is used to measure deep dose only

71.True regarding critical examination

a.carried out before use of equipment

b.concerned with radiation safety

c.installer responsible for critical examination

d.must be carried out in conjuction with RPA.

e.the RPA is appointed prior to installation

72.Principle recommendations in the Medical and Dental Guidance Notes is/are

a.leakage radiation from the tube should be less than 1mGy/hr ata distance of 1m from the focus

b.the total filtration of the tube and tube assembly should be less than the equivalent of 2.5mm of aluminium

c.the operator should stand at least 2 m from the tube

d.the housing and support plate for the image intensifier should have shielding of at least 2 mm lead equivalence.

e.skin entrance dose rates should not exceed 100 mGy /min

73.True regarding radiation exposure

a.more than 1mSv exposure in any year is noted in less than about 1% of staff whose dose is monitored

b.radiopharmacy staffs and interventional radiologist are among those receiving highest radiation

doses c.finger doses may approach 150 mSV /year to interventional radiologist doing biliary drainage.

d.The IRR99 only makes it mandatory to monitor the dose to classified staff

e.the monitoring period for classified staff would generally be 1months.

74.True regarding the IRR99

a.makes mandatory to monitor the dose to classified staff

b.HSE issue passbook for worker working with more than one radiation employer

c.HSE gives approval for the dosimeter service

d.the employer has responsibility for compliance with IRR99

e.the employer has responsibility to monitor doses to people working in controlled areas

75.Multiplying factor of 1.5 is applied to intended dose in case of

a.interventional radiology

b.radiographic and fluoroscopic involving contrast agents

c.nuclear medicine with intended effective dose >5mSv

d.CT examination

e.mammography

76.True regarding classified persons

a. are at no risk from ionization radiations

b.age 18 yrs or below

c.subject to dose monitoring

d.subjects to biennual health checks

e.health check-up records to be kept for 50 yrs beyond the dates the individual stop working as a classified person

77. True regarding film used as personal dosimeters

a. film is the traditional material of choice
b. has same emulsion on both side of film
c. degree of blackening of the film provide an indicator of dose
d. needs relatively simple equipment for processing and reading
e. provides permanent record of exposure

78. Incidents that are to be notified to HSE by the employer

a. an individual receiving a dose greater than any relevant dose limit
b. spliltting of a radiation source causing significant contamination
c. lost or stolen radiation source
d. loss of more than 200MBq of technetium -99
e. radiation dose much greater than intended

79. Phosphorescence differ from fluorescence

a. empty electron traps
b. a time delay in light emission (10^{-10}s to 10^{-3}s)
c. light emission facilitated by heating
d. used in radiology
e. used in grid

80. True regarding disadvantages of film as personal dosimeter

a. poor energy –dependence for sensitivity of the film
b. the overall sensitivity is no better than 0.5-1mSv
c. cannot be used for assessment of finger dose
d. subject to environmental effect such as heat
e. unsuitable for monitoring over periods greater than 1 months

81. True regarding thermoluminescent dosimeters (TLD)

a. no use of filters
b. can be reused for once
c. most common dosimeter used for assessment of finger dose
d. can be read once
e. minimal energy dependence for response

82. According to IRMER

a. the refferer initiates the x ray request
b. justification and authorization of procedure by the practitioner
c. the operator carries out the practical aspects of exposure following authorization
d. both the refferer and the practitioner must be healthcare pfofessionals
e. practitioner and operator must have adequate training in radiation protection

83. True regarding refferer in IRMER 2000

a. the employer define the entitlement of refferer and to provide referral criteria
b. the employer place no restriction on examination that may be requested
c. general practitioner may not be permitted to request for a CT scan
d. medical practitioner may be given automatic entitlement to be refferer
e. refferer is required to provide no clinical information

84. True regarding practitioner in IRMER 2000

a. role of justification of individual

exposure

b.require only practical experience in imaging to be designated as practitioner

c.authorisation is generally given by the IRMER practitioner

d.very broad role

e.never provide written justification

85.True regarding protection of the patients

a.proper collimation

b.use of magnified fields of view during fluoroscopy

c.keep the image intensifier as close as possible to the patients

d.removal of anti scatter grid on fluoroscopy

e.use of additional filters (generally cupper)

86.True regarding patients typical effective dose

a.CT abdomen or pelvis 10mSv

b.CT chest 8 mSv

c.barium enema 7 mSv

d.technetium -99m bone scan 4mSv

e.intravenous urogram 3mSv

87.True regarding Diagnostic reference levels

a.refers to doses for typical examinations for standard –sized patients

b.serve as aid to optimization

c.local DRL has nothing to do with national DRL

d.local DRL is set by the operator

e.DRL set in terms of measurable quantities such as dose area product

88.Healthcare practitioners who are generally entitiled to at as IRMER practitioner ai/are

a.radiologist

b.radiographers

c.dentists

d.cardiologists

e.ARSAC certificate holders.

89.Employee's procedure required by IRMER 2000 comprise

a.for diagnostic reference levels

b.medical research programmes

c.information to patients

d.for evaluation of a medical exposure and recording dose

e.to minimize the risk of accidental exposures

90.True regading MARS 1978

a.related with protection of patients

b.related with protection of population as a whole

c.ARSAC certificate is issued by IRMER

c.ARSAC issues guidance on approved tests

d.ARSAC issues guidance on normal and maximum levels of activity to be used

e.the license is specific to hospital

91.True regarding IRMER operator

a.very broad role

b.all practical aspects of the medical exposure that might affect patients dose or image quality

c.must be registered healthcare professional

d.service engineer is a operator

e.radiologist is a operator

92.Written procedures required by IRMER 2000 comprise

a.patients identification

b.entitlement to act as refferer ,practitioner,or operator

c.for medico-legal exposures

d.to establish about patients

pregnancy or breast feeding

e.for quality assurance programmes

93. True regarding patients typical effective dose

a.barium meal 2.5 mSv

b.CT head 2.0 mSv

c.barium swallow 1.5 mSv

d.technetium -99m lung perfusion study 1 mSv

e.lumbar spine (two film) 0.8 mSv

94.Radioactive Substances Act 1993 consists of

a.concerned with the protection of the population as a whole and the protection of the environment

b.provision for license or registration to hold radioactive sources

c.disposal through licensed disposal routes

d.regular inspection of hospital by the enforcing authorities

e.concerned with the protection of the patients

95.patients exposed to Low dose effective dose (<0.02mSv) comprise investigation of

a.chest PA view

b.shouder AP view

c.dental oraoral

d.extremities

e.pelvis AP

96.True regarding DRLs

a.generally set taking into account of dose audits

b.used to assess whether the dose for an individual is excessive

c.may be considered as the boundary between good and standard practice and poor abnormal practice

d.local DRL cannot be set in isolation

e.used to test wether average dose used for a particular examination is being restricted as far as reasonably practicable

97.True regarding TLD

a.barium fluoride is most common TLD material used as thermoluminescent material

b.the sensitivity of lithium fluoride is not strongly dependent on the X-ray spectrum

c.the atomic number of barium (8.2) is similar to that of tissue

d. TLD is heated to typically to 250 degree Celsius for reading

e.the measurement uncertainty using TLD is typically +/-5%

98.True regarding historical review of radioprotection

a.the first American radiation fatality in 1904 (death of Thomas Edison'assistant ,Clarence M Dolly)

b.the British X ray and Radiation protection committee founded in 1921 for recommendation to reduce radiation exposure

c.In 1928, Second International Congress of Radiology appointed committee to define Roentgen

d.first dose limiting recommendations was 0.2R/day

e.the National Council on Radition Protection and Measurement(NCRP) is a private organization

99.True regarding entrance surface dose

a.can be measured directly using TLD

b.for chest PA 0.12mGy

c.lumbar spine lateral 10 mGy

d.pelvis AP 3.2 mGy

e.skull AP or PA 1.9 mGy

100.True regarding RULE

a.justification of dose by the practitioner (IRMER)

b.doses kept ALARP and adherence to DRL by the operator (IRMER)

c.patient dose assessment to be part of the equipment quality assurance programme(IRR99)

d.DAP is becoming the most common quantity to use for patients dose audit

e.set DRL for representative examinations (IRMER)

101.True regarding radiation units

a.the roentgen is unit of radiation exposure

b.one roentgen liberate a charge of 2.56×10^{-4} coulombs/kg of air

c.the roentgen is dependent of area as a measure of exposure

d.the rad is unit of absorbed dose

e.one rad =the radiation necessary to deposit energy of 100 ergs in one kilogram of irradiated material

102.True regarding population exposures

a.effective dose equivalent is meant to relate exposure to risk

b.an effective dose equivalent of 0.06 mSv means that the risk involved from chest examination is the same as the risk involved in exposing the entire body to an xray exposure of 0.06mSv

c.the average cosmic annual dose equivalent is about 0.26 mSv (26mrem) at sea level

d.Cosmic radiation exposure approximately triples for each 2000-m increase in altitude

e.the average annual gamma ray effective dose equivalent is about 0.28 mSv(28 mrem)

103.True regarding source of radiation

a.major components of terrestrial gamma radiation are ^{40}k,members of thorium and uranium series

b.ingested radionuclides include ^{40}k,^{87}Rb,^{14}C, and members of the thorium and uranium series

c.inhaled radon is the largest contributor of the average annual effective dose equivalent

d.the estimated annual effective dose equivalent from radon sources is 2mSv

e.annual effective dose equivalent from **ingested radionuclides is 39 mrem**

104.True regarding supervised area

a.possibility of exposure to staff or the public

b.exposure conditions kept under review

c.may be conversion to controlled area in future

d.likelihood of exposure exceeding the dose limit for a member of the public (1 mSv/year)

e.the waiting room of patients injected with radiopharmaceutical agent

105.True regarding quality factor(Q)

a.Q is a function of particle type and energy

b.quality factor of X rays,Gamma rays ,Beta particles and Electrons is 1

c.quality factor of thermal neutronos is 5 while that of protons and alpha particles is 20

d.amount of biologic damage is

111

determined by the linear energy transfer (LET)of the radiation

e.protons is a higher energy LET radiation

106.IRMER 2000 concerns

a.justification and optimization of individual exposure

b.the responsibilities of the employer

c.diagnostic reference levels

d.medical physics expert

e.notification and enfocement

107.True regarding a nonstochastic effect of radiation exposure

a.somatic effect

b.effect increases with increasing absorbed dose

c.usually degenerative changes such as organ atrophy and fibrosis

d.example are lens opacification and decreased prem production

e. examples –cancers and genetic effects

108.True regarding protective barriers

a.primary barrier protect from primary radiation (the useful beam)

b.stray radiation refers to a scatter radiation only

c.the workload is the product of tube current in m A and time in minutes of exposure per week (m A-min/wk)

d.R/m A.min at 1 m at 125 kVp is 1.4

e.the use (U) factor (beam direction factor) for ceilings(useful beam) is always one

109.True regarding the protective barrier

a.the use factor is the fraction of time that the beam is detected at a particular barrier

b.the occupancy factor is expressed as a fraction that represents the amount of time that the area will be occupied

c.If effective weekly exposure reaching the point in question is greater than the maximal permissible exposures ,a protective barrier is required

d.concept of half-value layer (HVL) is used for calculating barrier requirement

e.attenuation curve is also used to calculate barrier requirement in diagnostic installation

110.True regarding sodium iodide (doped with thallium)

a.the traps generated are about 30 ev above the band of valence electrons

b.emitted photons is in invisible range

c.high stopping efficiency

d.rapid response time

e.thallium 01% by weight

111.True regarding radiation protection

a.the half value layer is thickness of a specific substance that reduce the exposure rate by one half

b. a beam with a HVL of 0.2mm of lead is less penetrating than a beam with a HVL of 0.1 mm of lead

c.HVL thickness for lead at 150 kVp is 0.09mm

d.filtration of x rays decrease HVL requirement

e.concrete may be used as primary and secondary barrier

112.Factors favouring using ionization and air for radiation measurement is /are

a.ionisation is an extremely sensitive process in terms of energy deposition

b.ionisation is related to extreme sensitivity of biological tissues to radiation

c.air is readily available

d.air compostion is close to being universally constant

e.atomic number of air(Z=7.6) is very close to that of muscle/soft tissue(Z=7.4)

113.True regarding free air ionization chamber

a.a primary standard for radiation measurement

b. more sensitive when compared to solid detectors

c.bulky in design

d.operates over very broad range of X-rays

e.accuracy better than 1% is required

114.True regarding Dosimetry.

a.Dose area product meters consists of flat ,large area parallel plate ionization chamber

b Bleeper worked on principle of modified Geiger-Muller principle

c.TLD needs to be heated for reading

d.high pressure xenon gas chamber is based on principle of ionization in gas

e.The fountain-pen dosimeter used the principle of gold leaf electroscope

115.True regarding the dose

a.the exit dose is typically between 0.1% to 1% of the entrance dose

b.the entrance surface dose is defined as the absorbed dose in air at the point of intersection of the x ray beam axis with the entrance surface of the patients including back scattered radiation

c.TLD generally provide the most straightforward and most accurate method of measurement of the entrance surface dose

d.indirect medthods of measuring the entrance surface dose is difficult to apply to automatic control systems

e.national reference dose for lumbar spine AP is 10 mGy

116.True regading energy levels in materials

a.the electrons in conduction band has sufficient energy to move freely through the crystalline materials

b.semiconductors has wide forbidden band

c.electron trap is localized discrete energy level close to the conduction band

d.hole trap is close to the valence band

e.the highest energy band is of valence band

117.Regarding optimization of radiation use

a.dose should be as low as reasonably achievable(ALARA principle)(IRCP)

b.take into account of economic and social factors

c.dose should be as low as reasonably practicable (ALARP principle)(UK phraseology)

d.design of equipment and selection of technique are part of optimization

e.operator technique and quality assurance programme are part of

optimization
118. True regarding ionization chamber
a.measure air kerma by measuring the amount of ionization produced by the photon beam in air

b.thimble chamber consisists of a thin central electrode

c.theoretically ,the air kerma is 34/mass of air in the chamber

d. a voltage applied between the outer thimble wall and the central electrode is typically in the range of 10-30 V

e.for each ion pair ,approximately 3 ev of energy is deposited

Answer
Radiation hazards and protection,Dosimetry, Uk Regulations

1.bd-----Measurement of X- rays and gamma rays is extremely difficult to measure absorbed dose in solids or liquids directly.Absorbed dose measurement by temperature rise is highly impractical.Conversion factor for bone is about 5 at low kev to 1.2 at 150 kev. Conversion factor for fat is about 0.6 at low kev to 1.1 at high kev. (page no.17 Farr).

2.abcde ---(page no.17 Farr).

3.abcd-----For diagnostic purposes .kerma and absorbed dose are equal.At high energies (greater than about 1Mev),they are different. The only practical difference between the two is that at high energies ,a small part of the energy of the electrons may produce bremstrahlung radiation,and the energy transferred to electrons at a specified location will be deposited away from that location because of the electron range. Kerma applies to x rays ,gamma rays and also neutrons. (page no.17 Farr).

4. bce ----- Ionization chamber may have any shape but commonest chambers are either cylindrical or consist of parallel electrodes .Chamber volume of approximately 10-30cm^3 are suitable for the measurement in the radiation beam with chambers of 150 or bigger being suitable for the measurement of scatter radiation. .
(page no/18 Farr).

5.abcde ---(page no/18 Farr).

6.bde---- In thimble chamber, the ionization current is measured by a device known as an electrometer.Correction for ambient temperature or pressure is small and is generally ignored---(page no.17 Farr).

7.ad----Chamber wall of thimble chamber must be made of air-equivalent material that matches air in terms of its effective atomic number plastic material is used as wall because its effective atomic number is 6 (effective atomic number of air 7.6).Graphite is deposited on inner wall to make it electrically conducting.Wall thickness of 0.2mm is sufficient for photoelectrons from 140 kev,however thinner wall chamber is used for mammography. ---(page no.18 Farr).

8.acd----Dose area product meters is meant for assessment of patients dose,mounted on the collimator of x ray tube .It uses of parallel plate type ionization chamber ,generally with square plate.The amount of ionization produced is proportional to dose and to the area of beam. ---(page no.18 Farr).

9.ac---intensity is greater for higher rather than low atomic number targets.The most complete description of quality is the spectrum of x ray energies.The greater is the HVL ,the greater the effective energy. ---(page no.19

Farr).

10.abcd---Luminescence can be divided into fluorescence and phosphorescence .there is instantaneous emission of light following energy input in fluorescence .There is delayed light emission (delay time of order of 10^{-6} s) in phosphorescence .Phosphor refers to a material that has luminescent properties.Scintillants are nothing but crystalline materials with luminescent properties that are used for the detection of gamma radiations.(page no.19 Farr).

11.abcde---(page no.20 Farr).

**12.abcde---- **---(page no.19 Farr).

13.abcde------(page no.19 Farr).

14.ace--- Conduction band remains vacant ,there is no electrons .Energy band of valence band<forbidden band<conduction band. ---(page no.20 Farr).

15.bc---- Impurities in phosphor is deliberatly introduced to create electron trap in the forbidden zone of the phosphor.The process of excitation raises electrons from the valence into the conduction band Electrons in the conduction band move freely within the material. (page no.20 Farr).

16.abcde---(page no.20 Farr).

17.ae--- Radiation damage is caused by radiation absorption .Chemical changes are produced virtually immediately ,and subsequent molecular damage follows in a short space of time (seconds to minutes).Biological damage becomes evident after much longer time of absorption (hours to decade) . ---(page no.23 Farr).

18.bc---- Impurities in phosphor is deliberatly introduced to create electron trap in the forbidden zone of the phosphor.The process of excitation raises electrons from the valence into the conduction band Electrons in the conduction band move freely within the material. ---(page no.20 Farr).

19.abcde---(page no.20 Farr).

20.ce---beta particle in tissue follow a very tortuous path because beta partcicles are easily deflected by orbital electrons of tissue.Total range involved in tissue interaction is of the order of a few millimeters. Beta particle eventually gives all its energy to tissue.Unlike beta particles x ray and gamma rays radiations donot have a maimum depth of penetration associated with them ,but they simply undergo progressive attenuation,that is the intensity of the radiation beam continues to fall as it interacts with tissue but at any give depth a residual beam always remains. ---(page no.23-24 Farr).

21.abcde---(page no.11 Farr).

22.abde---- The hydroxyl free radical is highly reactive and powerful oxidizing agent. (page no.24 Farr).

23.ace----Linearity of response is noted in TLD ,not in film badge.TLD response is independent of TLD except at low kv. ---(page no.325 Farr).

24.abe--- Electron is a low-LET radiation than that of alpha particle.Damage caused by high-LET radiation is more likely to be non-repairable because ionizing events caused by high-LET are much more closely spaced and within diastances comparable with the dimentions of a single strand of DNA. ---(page no.24 Farr).

25.abcde-------(page no.26 Farr).

26.ade---- deterministic effect on lens is cumulative and has no repair mechanism. ---(page no.26Farr).

27.ab ---Deterministic effect has threshold dose ,but there is small variation in threshold from individual to individual.Most deterministic effect have repair mechanisms ,except damage to eye.The greatest fetal abnormality is seen in the third week to eigth week of pregnancy. ---(page no.25-26 Farr).

28.abd---absorbed dose is independent of the composition of the radiated material and energy of the beam.Rad is unit of absorbed dose.(Page 374/ Christensen].

29.abcde----- The more rapidly a cell is dividing ,greater is its sensitivity(law of Bergonie and Tribondeau)
(page 280/P P Dendy)

30.abc----rem=rads x quality factor.Quality factor for x rays is 1.(page no.374Farr).

31.abcde---(page no.26 Farr).

32.ade---- Risk factor for the thyroid cancer is relatively low because ,although the probability of induction is relatively high,mortality is low .Overall ,for a uniform whole body irradiation,the risk of fatal cancer is 5% per Sv or 1 in 20000 per mSv for general population. ---(page no.27 Farr).

33.abcd---a CT scan of pelvis during pregnancy will double the risk of fatal childhood cancer. (page no.28 Farr).

34.ace----- In stochastic effect of radiation exposure, the severity of the effect doesnot depend on the magnitude of the absorbed dose,there is no dose threshold. ---(page no.377 Farr).

35.abcde---(page no.29 Farr).

36.abcde---(page no.27 Farr).

37.abd----Tissue weighting factor assigned to gonad is 0.2.The sum of weighting factors is 1. ---(page no.17-28 Farr).

38.acd----DAP can be easily measured ,can be converted to effective dose using conversion factor Conversion factor used is not fixed .depend on region of body examined ,on projection and also on Kv and beam filtration. ---(page no.45-46 Farr).

39.abcde---(page no.29 Farr).

40.bcd----No secondary barrier is required for areas protected by a primary barrier.The energy of secondary radiation is assumed to be equal to that of the primary radiation (Page 383-90/Christensen].

41.bde----All ionizing radiation are harmful.latent period for leukaemia range from 5 to 20 yrs and from 10 to 30 yrs for other tumours (Page 383-90/Christensen].

42.abcde-------(page no.37 Farr).

43.cde----- Electronic dosimeters are direct reading device,so very useful in identifying methods of dose reduction for procedures in which there is the potential for high doses to the staff,and for teaching. Response is highly energy-dependent ,but if placed behind suitable filters they can provide reasonably accurate dose measurements down to 20 keV. --- (page no.37 Farr).

44.ade---- Thermoluminescent dosimeters (TLD) has minimal energy dependence for response and its overall sensitivity is not significantly better than film.(page no.37 Farr).

45.abcde---(page 136/ P P Dendy)

46.abcde--- (page no.29/Farr)

47.abcde---- (page no.29/Farr)

48.acd---cosmic radiation is a mixture of particulate radiation and a broad spectrum of X- and gamma rays.The cosmic radiation increases with altitude,so air travelers receive approximately 4micoSv/hour due to the reduced effect of attenuation in the atmosphere. (page no.29/Farr)

49.abcde-----(page no.29/Farr)

50.abcde----(page no.30/Farr)

51.ace ---The Health and Safety at Work Act (1974) established an advisory body ,the Health and Safety Commission(HSC) ,and the Health and Safety Executive (HSE) and this regulations are part of the criminal law,HSE has power of inspection and prosecution. (page no.31/Farr)

52.abcde---(page no.29/Farr)

53.abcde-----(page no.24/Farr)

54.abd----Direct radiation damage is due to rupture of covalent bonds in the solute molecules.Indirec radiation damage is more comman than direct radiation damage because living tissue is about 70-90 %.(page no.24/Farr)

55.abcde-----(page no.29/Farr)

56.abc----- HSC have published the three documents— IRR99,ACOP,and Guidance for good pactice.Guidance for good pactice has lesser status than the ACOP.The IRR99 is not concerned with the radiation protection of patients ,it is Ionising Radiation (Medical exposure) Regulations 2000(IRMER) that is concerned with radiation protection of patients . (page no.31/Farr)

57.abde----In the health service ,the RPA is almost invariably a medical physicist. (page no.31/Farr)

58.abcde-----(page no.32/Farr)

59.abd---Barium plaster is one of protective material which exploits the photoelectric effect by substituting barium with its high atomic number for calcium in standard plaster.Viewing window is made of lead glass .
(page no.41/Farr)

60.abcde----(page no.41/Farr)

61.ace---Overcouch screening table are not suitable for interventional studies.Barium and tin is incorporated in lead apron to reduce the weight of apron.Lead apron of 0.25mm,0.35mm,0.5mm transmit approximately 5%,3%and 1.5% respectively.Amajor issue of use of apron is discomfort.The weight of the apron can be reduced by having thinner lead on the back and also by use of light weight materials such as barium and tin .Barium and tin has K-edges in the mid to lower part of the X-rays with energies below the

K-edge of lead (88keV) (page no.43/Farr)

62.ade----The film badge holder contains a number of filters which extend the range of radiation energies and aslso provide data which may be used to calculate the dose for low energies photons and electrons. cadmium filter.Cadmium filter capture neutrons with subsequent emission of gamma rays so additional blackening under the filter is evidence of neutron. (page no.323-24/Farr)

63.abd---True regading pregnant staff,fetal dose is equal to the dose monitoring reading in radionuclide imaging .Fetal dose is equal 50% of the dose monitoring reading in X-ray imaging . (page no.32/Farr)

64. ade----Ionization chamber and Geiger-Muller counters, both respond to x-ray and gamma rays and to fast beta particles. Because of internal amplification ,the GM tube is more sensitive than than the ionization chamber.The inonisation chamber is designed to collect all primary and secondary radiation and hence to give a reading of exposure or exposure rate.With the GM tube there is no proportional relationship between the count rate and the number of primary and secondary ionizations ,so it is not a radition monitor. (page 141/ P P Dendy)

65.ab-----Acoording to IRR99 ,dose relaxation cannot be applied to employees, parent holding young child for x ray position is not comforters and carers,comforter and carers areexpalained the risk involved (Chapter 2,page

no.32,second edition (page no./Farr)

66.bde----The effective dose limit is concerned with carcinogenic risk.The dose limits for employees(16-18yrs) is three-tenths of that set for employees above 18 yrs or above. (page no.32/Farr)

67.acde----In controlled areas ,likely to get exposure greater than three-tenths of any dose limit. (page no.32/Farr)

68.abde--- For mobile x ray equipment ,designation of the whole room as controlled area is generally impractical and it is standard practice to designate the area within 2m of the X-ray tube and patients as the controlled area. (page no.33/Farr)

69.acde----Local rules are written instructions for people working in controlled or supervised areas(page no.33/Farr)

70. acd---- the personal dose equivalent at a depth of 10mm is reffered as the deep dose .The standard body badge is used to measure both deep dose and the shallow dose and so includes filters so that an estimate of radiation energy to which the person has been exposed can be made and for the two quantities to be calculated (page no.37/Farr)

71.abcd--- RPA is not necessarily appointed by the installer prior to installation. (page no.34/Farr)

72.abcde---- (page no.35/Farr)

73.abcde---(page no.35/Farr)

74.abcde----(page no.35-36/Farr)

75.abcd----Multiplying factor of 10 is applied to intended dose in case of mammography, nuclear medicine with intended effective dose < 5mSv . Multiplying factor of 20 is applied to intended dose in case of radiography of extremities ,skull,dentition,shoulder,chest ,elbow and nuclear medicine with intended effective dose < 0.5mSv. (page no.37/Farr)

76.ce----Staffs designed as classified persons are at risk from ionization radiations,are of age of 18 yrs or above and are certified as being medically fit to work as a classified person (by doctor appointed by HSE),are subject to dose monitoring and subjects to annual health check-up----(page no.34/Farr)

77.acde-- Film used as personal dosimeters has different emulsion on each side of the film with different sensitivities.The fast (most sensitive) emulsion is used routinely ,but if the badge has received a particularlyhigh dose it will be too black to providea meaningful result.This emulsion can then be removed and the less sensitive side of the film is used to extent the useful range of the badge. (page no.36/Farr)

78.abce---Incidents that are to be notified to HSE by the employer includes loss of more than 100MBq of technetium -99 (page no.37/Farr)

79.abcd---- (page 84-85/ P P Dendy)

80.cde---- The sensitivity of the film (optical density as a function of dose) is highly energy dependent because of the high atomic numbers of silver and bromine in the emulsion.The overall sensitivity is no better than 0.1-0.2mSv. dosimeter(page no.36-37/Farr)

81.cde----Thermoluminescent dosimeters (TLD) are used in conjunction with filters set in the badge holder no use of filters and can be reused for once . (page no.37/Farr)

82.abcde---(page no.37/Farr)

83. acd----- IRMER 2000,the employer may place restriction on examination that may be requested .Refferer is required to provide sufficient clinical information for the IRMER practitioner to be best able to determine whether the examination is justified. (page no.38/Farr)

84.ac---Practitioner in IRMER 2000 require both theoretical knowledge of radiation protection and imaging and practical experience in the specific area of clinical practice ,has a single role of justification of individual exposures .The IRMER practitioner may provide written justification guidelines to permit the operator to authorize an examination in particular clinical circumstances. (page no.39/Farr)

85.abcde---(page no.43/Farr)

86.abcde----(page no.44/Farr)

87.abe-----L ocal DRL is set by the employer and reflect local practice.In general,this is through patients dose audit.In setting the local DRL ,it is a requirement to take account of national or European DRLs.The local value should not be greater than the national DRL unless it can be justified on clinical grounds. (page no.40/Farr)

88.abcde---- (page no.39/Farr)

89.abcde--- (page no.39/Farr)

90.acde---Under MARS 1978 ----- the ARSAC certificate is issued by a committee ARSAC (page no.41/Farr)

91.abce---IRMER doesnot require the operator to be registered healthcare professional . (page no.39/Farr)

92.abcde----(page no.39/Farr)

93.abcde---(page no.44/Farr)

94.abcd---(page no.41/Farr)

95.abcd------(page no.44/Farr)

96.acde---(page no.45-46/Farr)

97.bde----Lithium fluoride is most common TLD material used as thermoluminescent material,the atomic number of lithium (8.2) is similar to that of tissue.
(page no.44/Farr)

98.abcde----
True regarding historical review of radioprotection----
(page no.372/Farr)

99.abcde----(page no.45/Farr)

100.abcde--- (page no.45/Farr)

101.abd----The roentgen is independent of area as a measure of exposure.one rad =the radiation necessary to deposit energy of 100 ergs in 1gram of irradiated material---(page no.373-74/Farr)

102.abce---
Cosmic radiation exposure approximately doubles for each 2000-m increase in altitude.(Page 375/ Christensen].

103.abcde----.(Page 375/ Christensen].

104. abcde ---.(Page 33/ Christensen]

105.abcde---.(Page 375/ Christensen].

106.abcde—.(Page 37/ Farr].

107.abce-------.(Page 377/ Christensen].

108.acd----primary barrier protect from primary radiation (the useful beam) while secondary barrier protect from stray radiation (combination of leakage and scatter radiation).The use (U) factor (beam direction factor) for ceilings(useful beam) is always zero(0).U for secondary barrier is always 1. ---.(Page 371-81/ Christensen].

109.abcd ---Attenuation curve is used to calculate barrier requirement in therapeutic installation---.(Page 380-82/ Christensen].

110.cd---- In Sodium iodide (doped with 0.1% by weight thallium), the traps generated are about 3 ev above the band of valence electrons and emitted photons is in visible range---.(Page 147/ Christensen].

111.ae--- A beam with a HVL of 0.2mm of lead is more penetrating than a beam with a HVL of 0.1 mm of lead.HVL thickness for lead at 150 kVp is 0.29mm.Filtration of x rays increase HVL requirement ---.(Page 382-83/ Christensen].

112.abcde------ (page 136/ P P Dendy)

113.ace----- Free air ionization chamber is insensitive when compared to solid detectors,operates over only a limited range of X-rays because secondary electrons produced especiall above 300 keV. ------ (page 136/ P P Dendy)

114.abcde---------- (page 143-46/ P P Dendy)

115.abcde--------- (page 155-57/ P P Dendy)

116.acd----Semiconductors has narrow forbidden band .The highest energy band is of conduction band------ (page 83-85/ P P Dendy)

117.abcde---------- (page 30/ Farr)

118.abc---Thimble chamber consisists of a plastic thimble-shaped outer wall surrounding an air- filled cavity and a central electrode.Each x-ray photon absorbed in the wall liberate a secondary electron which produces ion pairs along its track.For each ion pair,approximately 34 ev of energy is deposited.A voltage applied between the outer thimble wall and the central electrode is typically in the range of 100-300 V and is meant to separate ions before they can recombine. . (page 30/ Farr)

CHAPTER 7
Digital Radiography

1.True regarding analogue and digital image
a.a direct spatial relationship between the X-ray photons and the response of recording medium
b.developed photographic film is an example of an analogue image
c. easy to extract quantitative data from an analogue image
d.x ray interaction is assigned to appropriate compartments (pixel) in digital data
e.he number and size of pixels are fixed in digital imaging

2.True regarding Digital imaging
a.image storage size is important due to computer memory,archive capacity and for processing time and in transmission time
b.in lossless /reversible compression,the image can be restored into an identical version of the original
c.in lossy /irreversible compression,the displayed image doesnot perfectly reproduce the original
d.lossless compression allows greater reduction of image storage size than lossy compression
e. lossy compression allows reduction of image storage size upto about 5 times

3.True regarding digital image
a.the digitized image is essentially a matrix of numbers
b.a certain brightness level is assigned to all numbers within a particular range
c.the detector system must record x -ray quanta with a high efficiency
d.the detector system must be capable of providing with spatial information about the distribution of X-rays
e.there is greater dynamic range of of digital image

4.True regarding digital imaging
a.the image is divided into a matrix of individual cells or pixels
b.each pixel has variable value
c.pixel with low value are displayed as dark
d.the matrix size ,the pixel size and field of view are all interrelated
e.pixel size =matrix size /field of view

5.True regarding pixel .
a.pixel size is related to spatial resolution
b.usually objects smaller than the dimensions of a pixel is routinely seen
c.the value stored in each pixel is stored in binary format
d.the minimum value that is stored is related to the bit depth of the pixel
e.the greater the bit depth ,greater is the potential to display contrast

6.True regarding bit and byte
a.a single bit store images only as either black or white
b.a 12-bit pixel has 4096 levels of grey
c.a byte can carry up to 8 bits(a

number up to a value of $2^8-1 = 255$)
d.computer memory is expressed in terms of the number of bytes
e.the greater the bit depth ,the greater is the potential to display contrast

7.True regarding cathode ray tube image display
a.the cathode ray tube utilizes a scanning electron beam
b.intensity of scanning electron beam is modulated in accordance with the stored pixel values
c.typically ,there are upto 1250 scan lines
d.the resolution perpendicular l to the scan lines is limited by the frequency of the modulating signal
e.the resolution in the parallel to the scan lines is limited by number of scan lines

8.True regarding radiography
a.the maximum matrix size is largely determined by the imaging modality
b.conventional radiography has high intrinsic spatial resolution($10 lp mm^{-1}$)
c.DR systems need small matrix sizes
d.radionuclide images has low level of noises
e.in DR,detectors have a very norrow dynamic range

9.True regarding digital imaging
a.the image is divided into a matrix of individual cells or pixels
b.each pixel has variable value
c.pixel with low value are displayed as dark
d.the matrix size ,the pixel size and field of view are all interrelated
e.pixel size =matrix size / field of view

10.True regarding image display.
a.liquid crystal display is a kind of flat –panel monitor
b.calibration is an important feature of the image display
c.there is no standard in display calibration in DICOM
d.the standard takes into account of perceptivity of the human eye and ear both
e.subject to quality assurance – programme

11.True regarding Fourier analysis.
a.help to understand the performance of imaging system
b.here the image signal is broken down into a series of sine waves that vary in terms of spatial frequency and amplitude
c.small,sharp structure is composed of high spatial frequencies
d.used in reconstructionof image in CT
e.used in reconstruction of image in MRI and USG

12.True regarding noise
a.in fluoroscopy ,noise can be reduced by adding the signal from successive frames to give a time-averaged image
b.frame averaging is useful when there is no movement between frames
c.noise may be reduced by low-pass spatial filtering
d.noise may be reduced by edge enhancement or high –pass filtering
e.low-pass filter may generate false structures in the image

13.True regarding CR and DR
a. CR system involve removing the cassette from X-ray set, taking the

plate to a reader and waiting for a period for about 1min

b.DR systems use imaging devices that remain in situ

c.DR systems produce an image with a delay that is generally no more than about 1 min

d.DR systems use photostimulable phosphors

e.The most CR detectors are based on amorphous silicon thin-film transistor (TFT) arrays

14.True regarding sampling to avoid aliasing

a.the signal must be sampled at least twice in every cycle or period(The Nyquist criteria)

b.the sampling frequency must be at least twice the highest frequency present in the signal

c.the maximum signal frequency that can be accurately sampled is called the Nyquist frequency

d.the Nyquist frequency is equal to half of the sampling frequency

e.in case of aliasing ,high frequency signals are recorded as low

15.True regarding Modulation transfer function

a.an objective method for comparing the imaging performance of different system

b.the ratio of the output/input modulation

c.MTF varies with spatial frequency ,generally reducing with increase of spatial frequency

d.Fourier analysis is used to assess MTF

e.MTF is used to analyse aliasing

16.True regarding imaging plates in computed radiography

a.use of calcium fluorohalide doped

with europium as potostimulable phosphor

b.halide in photostmulable phosphor is a combination of bromide and iodide,typically 85% and 15%

c.the plate is inserted into a light-tight cassestte

d.the potostimulable phosphor requires light input to release the trapped energy

e.most of phosphors used for CR emit light at blue end of spectrum

17.True regarding Aliasing artefact

a.low frequency streak artefact in CT

b.wrap-round in MRI

c.fast flow in one direction will be interpreted as slower flow in opposite direction in USG

d.aliasing is due to oversampling

e.The Nyquist criteria useful to understand aliasing

18.True regarding CR reader

a.plate is removed from cassette in reader and scanned by laser

b.optical fibre above the plate is used for scanning

c.rotating mirror above the plate direct emitted light to photomultiplier tubes

d.single scanning is enough to extract information

e.exposure of plate to light done to erase the residual signal

19.True regarding computed radiography

a.photostimulable phosphor have norrow dynamic range

b.there is a linear relationship between signal from a computed radiography plate and dose to the

125

plate

c.the latitude of the CR system is very much greater than for conventional radiography

d.choice of gradation curve are dependent on the projection

e.histogram analysis involves an analysis of the distribution of the light intensities outside the collimated area

20.True regarding imaging reader

a.most of CR phosphor need scanning laser emitting red light for stimulation

b.the time for a CR reader to extract the image from the plate is generally between 30-45s

c.in stacking readers ,several cassette may be placed in a queue for automatic feed

d.the residual signal after reading is left as such

e.roating mirror is to visualize the plate in the reader

21.True regarding spatial resolution

a.CR system show better spatial resolution than conventional radiography

b.CR system display more image contrast than that of film screen radiography

c.the typical spatial resolution of 7.7Mpixels matrix size is 3.5lp mm^{-1}

d.the typical spatial resolution of film screen radiography is 8 lp mm^{-1}

e.thin phosphor layer and crystalline structure degrades the spatial resolution of CR system

22.True regarding CCD-based digital detectors

a.used in conjunction with phosphor to detect the X-rays

b.cannot be manufactured in a size that is very much greater than 5 cm^2

c.used in mammography for stereotactic films used for biopsy localization

d.system is built with tiled array of CCDs to cover the full field required in radiography

e.detector with tiled array of CCDs are necessary for mammographic biopsy localization

23.True regarding detector dose indicators(DDIs)

a.DDIs are analogous to optical density of film

b.DDI is determined from the signal from the plate averaged over a broad region

c.DDI defintion is well defined and universally acceptable

d.manufacturers provide normal ranges for DDI

e.help to ensure the patients s dose as low as reasonably practicable

24.True regarding amorphous silicon thin-film transistor (TFT) arrays

a.TFT is essentially a large integrated circuit

b.the dimensions of array correspond to the size of the area to be imaged

c.a transistor is a device that minimize an electrical signal

d. in TFT, the amplified signal is stored as an electrical charge

e.The charge can be released by a high potential and is applied column by column

25.True regarding flat plate detector (indirect DR)

a.a phosphor convert X-ray photons

126

to light

b.the light is detected by photodiodes

c.calcium iodide and gadolinium oxysulphide are used as phosphor

d.calcium iodide is used in ward radiography

e.gadolinium oxysulphide is cheaper to produce and more robust

26.True regarding caesium iodide used in digital radiography

a.used as phosphor in direct digital radiography

b.crystalline phosphor oriented perpendicular to the surface of the detector

c.phosphor size diameter very much larger than the pixel size

d.relatively thick layer of phosphor used to increase the detection efficiency

e.internal reflection of light in the crystal

27.True regarding detector for direct digital radiography

a.amorphous selenium detector is used as a photoconductor

b.an X-ray photon interact in the photoconductor material and produces negative and positive charges

c.the upper surface of photoconductor is bonded to an electrode connected to a high positive potential

d.the negative charges are drawn to the charge collectors in the TFT array

e.charge is deposited on the amorphous silicon TFT as a single layer of material

28.True regarding TFT

a.each row of detectors is connected to the activating potential and each column to a charge-measuring device

b. in a TFT array,there are as many transistors as there are pixels

c.the size of each transistor ,or pixel is in range of 100-200micrometer

d.the electroncs and the detectors are deposited in several layers on a glass substrate

e.an X-ray or light detector is deposited above the charge collection device on the plate

29.True regarding spatial resolution in CR system

a.smaller pixel size has better spatial resolution

b.finer detail can be detected in CR with thinner phosphor

c.mammography uses thinner phosphor

d.finer detail detection can be improved by the partial volume effect

e. finer detail detection can be improved by the use of edge enhancement algorithms

30.True regarding digital radiography

a. Detective quantum efficiency (DOE) reflects the efficiency of phosphor detection and noise added to the detector signal

b.DQE may be 100% in DR system

c.DQE of CR system and film-screen system is close to 30%

d.Disadvantage of DR in comparison to CR are cost and versatility

e.a DR system have the same flexibility in positioning as a CR plate

31.Factors that govern the choice of suitable matrix size is/are

a.resolution cannot be better than the size of an individual matrix matrix element or pixel

b.the pixel size is governed by the field of view

c.a finer pixellation will improve resolution but place burden on computer in terms of data storage and manipulation

d.decreasing pixel size below the resolving capacity of the imaging equipment is of no use

e.as the pixel size becomes smaller ,the size of the signal becomes smaller and so the S/N ratio

32.True regarding computed radiography

a. The phosphor plate has a more linear response than the sigmoid-shaped curve of the film/screen combination

b. Photostimulable phosphor plates have anarrower latitude than film/screen.

c. a reduction in the number of repeat images in comparison to film

d. The spatial resolution of film is lower (approximately 2½ line-pairs per mm) than that of CR (approximately 5 line-pairs per mm

e. superior contrast resolution than to film

33.True regarding direct digital radiography

a.the amorphous silicon is used to make plates consisting of an array of photodiodes/transistors

b.caesium iodide or rare earth scintillators (detector) emit light photons

c. selenium detector produces an electrical signal

d. the amorphous silicon amplify the incoming light or electrical signal

e. The detector plates are fragile, heavy and fixed

34.True regarding direct digital radiography

a. The spatial resolution of direct DR is better than that of film

b. Direct DR has better detective quantum efficiency (DQE) than film

c. dose reduction per exposure than film

d. better contrast resolution than film

e.unlike photostimulable phosphor plates, a direct digital signal is produced

35.True regarding PACS

a. The British Royal College of Radiologists recommend of lossy compression for a definitive diagnostic report

b. Lossless compression techniques can currently achieve a maximum compression ratio of 30:1

c. Lossy compression techniques irreversibly compress the image and data are permanently lost,

d. The main requirement for image data compression arises in connection with teleradiology

e. lossy compression algorithm are joint photographic expert group (JPEG) compression, and wavelet compression

Answer
Digital Radiography

1.abd----It is not easy to extract quantitative data from an analogue image.The number and size of pixels are variable in digital imaging(64 x64 to 2048 x 2048) (page 193/ Dendy)

2.abc----Lossy compression allows greater reduction of image storage size than lossless compression.Lossy compression allows reduction of image storage size upto about 40 times. (page 80/ Farr)

3.abcde---- (page 193-94/ Dendy)

4.ade---In digital imaging, the image is divided into a matrix of individual cells or pixels.Each pixel has an assigned value that is related to the intensity of signal in the corresponding part of the image.Like conventional radiography ,the pixels having high values is displayed dark and those with low values is displayed as light.(page 79/ Farr)

5.ace---Pixel size is related to spatial resolution because objects smaller than the dimensions of a pixel will not be seen unless there is a very high degree of objects contrast,in which case the partial volume effect make it visible.The maximum value that is stored in pixel is related to the bit depth of the pixel .The greater the bit depth ,greater is the potential to display contrast. . (page 80/ Farr)

6.abcde----(page 80/ Farr)

7.abc---The resolution parallel to the scan lines is limited by the frequency of the modulating signal.The resolution in the perpendicular direction is limited by number of scan lines. (page 81/ Farr)

8.ab----- DR systems need large matrix sizes.Radionuclide images has high level of noises.In DR ,detectors have a very wide dynamic range. (page 80/ Farr)

9.ade---In digital imaging, the image is divided into a matrix of individual cells or pixels.Each pixel has an assigned value that is related to the intensity of signal in the corresponding part of the image.Like conventional radiography ,the pixels having high values is displayed dark and those with low values is displayed as light. (page 79/ Farr)

10.abe---Calibration is an important feature of the image display.There is a standard in display calibration in DICOM and that standard takes into account of perceptivity of the human eye. . (page 81/ Farr)

11.abcde ----(page 81/ Farr)

12.abc---- Edge enhancement or high –pass filtering increase the noise because such filter adds in a proportion of the difference between the grayscale value of the pixel and that of its neibhours.The effect is to exaggerate the contrast at the boundary between structures more visible .It may generate false structures in the image when a high level filtering is applied. (page 81/ Farr)

13.abc----CR systems use photostimulable phosphors.The most DR detectors are based on amorphous silicon thin-film transistor (TFT) arrays.The DR itself is divided into main classes :indirect DR and direct DR (DDR).) (page 86/ Farr)

14.abcde----(page 81/ Farr)

15.abcd----(page 83/ Farr)

16.bcde---- Imaging plates in computed radiography uses of barium fluorohalide doped with europium as potostimulable phosphor. (page 84/ Farr)

17.abce ----aliasing is due to undersampling (page 82/ Farr)

18.ae-----In CR reader, plate is removed from cassette in reader and scanned by laser .Rotating mirror is used for scanning.Optical fibres above the plate, direct emitted light to photomultiplier tubes.Repeated scanning is done to extract information. . (page 84/ Farr)

19.bce----Photostimulable phosphor have a wide dynamic range,being able to record photon intensities varying by a factor of about 10000:1.To display useful image ,the processing of the data from the reader involves to detect the collimated edges of the X-ray beam ,histogram analysis and optimization of gradation curve . Histogram analysis involves an analysis of the distribution of the light intensities within the collimated area. (page 84-85/ Farr)

20.abc---The residual signal after reading is erased by exposing to a bright light.The rotating mirror is used to scan the plate . (page 84/ Farr)

21.bcd----CR system has less spatial resolution than conventional radiography.The spatial resolution of CR system is influenced by the matrix size,phosphor thickness ,diameter od scanning laser and crystalline nature of phosphor .thin phosphor layer and crystalline structure improves the spatial resolution of CR system.(page 85/ Farr)

22.abcde----(page 87-88/ Farr)

23.abde----Detector dose indicators(DDIs)defintion is manufacturer –dependent.(such as the DDI is inversely proportional to dose,DDIs are functions of the dose) (page 86/ Farr)

24.abd------True regarding amorphous silicon thin-film transistor (TFT) arrays transistor is a device that amplifies an electrical signal and in TFT, the amplified signal is stored as an electrical charge.The charge can be released by a high potential and is applied row by row,so that timing of the detected signal determines the position of the pixel from which it originated. (page 86/ Farr)

25.abe---In flat plate detector (indirect DR), caesium iodide and gadolinium oxysulphide are used as phosphor.Gadolinium oxysulphide is used in ward radiography because it is cheaper to produce and more robust. (page 87/ Farr)

26.bde---- Caesium iodide is used as

phosphor in direct digital radiography .Phosphor size diameter is very much smaller than the pixel size. (page 87/ Farr)

27.abce---The positive charges are drawn to the charge collectors in the TFT array . (page 87/ Farr)

28.abcde-----(page 86/ Farr)

29.abcde.----- (page 85/ Farr)

30.acd---Detective quantum efficiency (DOE) reflects the efficiency of phosphor detection and noise added to the detector signal. DQE for DR system may be as high as 65%.DQE are lower than 100% because of less than 100% absorption of X-rays in the device and internal sources of noise. (page 87/ Farr)

31.abcde-----(page 193-94/ Dendy)

32.ace---- Photostimulable phosphor plates have a wider latitude than film/screen. The spatial resolution of CR is lower (approximately 2½ line-pairs per mm) than that of film (approximately 5 line-pairs per mm.(Chapter 1 Adam: Grainger)

33.abcde----(Chapter 1 ,Adam: Grainger)

34.bcde----The spatial resolution of direct DR equals that of film.(Chapter 1 ,Adam: Grainger.)

35.de----The British Royal College of Radiologists recommend of lossless compression for a definitive diagnostic report.Lossless compression techniques can currently achieve a maximum compression ratio of 3:1. As the name implies, lossless compression reversibly compresses the data so that no data are permanently lost from the image. .(Chapter 1 ,Adam: Grainger)

CHAPTER 8
Gamma Imaging

1. True regarding radionuclide images

a. depict organ function rather than organ structure

b. indicate the mapping of administered radiopharmaceutical in the body

c. radiation emitted within the body

d. biological behavior of radiopharmaceutical not important

e. depict cells and tissues too small for anatomical imaging

2. True regarding Gallium - 67

a. cyclotron produced

b. half-life of 78 hrs

c. decays by internal conversion

d. emit gamma rays of three energies (93,185,and 300 keV)

e. used to detect tumours and abscesses as it binds to fat

3. True regarding isotopes of carbon

a. all have six protons

b. carbon -11 ,carbon -14 are artificially produced

c. carbon -12 ,carbon -13 and carbon -14 are unstable and radioactive

d. carbon-11 has neutron excess

e. carbon -14 has neutron deficit

4. True regarding iodine -131

a. first radionuclide used for imaging

b. cheap ,highly reactive

c. produced in reactor

d. short half-life

e. emits gamma rays only

5. True regarding nuclei

a. nearly all nuclei extant unstable

b. ordinar hydrogen has single proton

c. the stable lighter nuclei has nearly equal number of protons and neutrons

d. the nucleus of helium atom is known as an beta particle

e. an alpha paricle has two neutrons and two protons and is unstable

6. True regarding radionuclide imaging

a. ^{99m}Tc sulphur colloid taken up by Küpfer cells

b. ^{99m}Tc HIDA taken up and excreted by hepatocytes

c. Leucocytes labelled (ex-vivo) using ^{99m}Tc HMPAO

d. Uptake of ^{18}F-FDG on PET due to increased expression of glucose transporters and hexokinase in breast carcinoma

e. Uptake and retention of ^{99m}Tc methoxyisobutylisonitrile on gamma scintigraphy dependent on perfusion and expression of multidrug resistance p-glycoprotein in breast carcinoma

7. True regarding atom

a. Rutherford established that atom has nucleus surrounded with electrons

b. Bohr Model support of electron in discrete orbits

c. Protons and neutrons are nearly 2000 times heavier than electrons,

d. A radionuclide is a nuclide that is radioactive.

e A radioactive nucleus is unstable and spontaneously disintegrate or decay at some time

8. Naturally occurring

radionuclides is/are
a.uranium
b.radium
c.radon
d.potassium-40
e.carbon-14

9.True regarding radionuclides
a.unstable nuclei having a neutron excess or deficit
b.more than 2700 known radionuclides
c.spontaneous transformation (or decay)
d.emit alpha,beta and gamma radiation
e.carbon-14 is naturally occurring radionuclides

10.True regarding production of radionuclides in nuclear reactor
a.additional neutron is forced into a stable nucleus making it unstable (neutron excess)
b.the atomic number of the nucleus remains unchanged
c.mass number of the nucleus increased by one
d.radionuclides produced can be seprated from the original stable nuclide
e.radionuclide produced can be made carrier free

11.True regarding cyclotron
a.accelerates postitively charged ion (protons,deuterons or alpha particle)
b.additinal protons are forced into a stable nucleus and neutralize neutron
c.produce nucleus with neutron excess
d.no change in the mass number of the nucleus
e.increase in atomic number

12.True regarding radionuclide
produced in a cyclotron
a.can be obtained carrier- free
b.can be seprated chemically from the original stable nuclides
c.short half-life (less than a minute to a couple of hours)
d.possible to use close to cyclotron only
e.F-18 can be produced by medical minicyclotrons

13.True regarding artificial method of radionuclide production
a.$^{98}Mo + n ---> ^{99}Mo$(nuclear reactor)
b.$^{18}o + p ---> ^{18}F + n$ (cyclotron)
c.$^{238}U ---> ^{98}Mo$ + other fission by-products(from spent fuel products of nuclear reactors)
d.$^{99}Tc^m$ from molybdenum - 99/$^{99}Tc^m$ generator
e.^{68}gallium from a gemanium-68 ($^{68}Ge/^{68}Ga$) generator

14.True regarding beta decay
a.seen in radionuclides with a neutron deficit
b.neutron changes into a proton plus positron
c.positron is ejected from the nucleus with high energy
d.decay of iodine -131 to xenon-131 is an example
e.no change of mass number but atomic number increases

15.True regarding isomers
a.different mass number
b.different number of protons and neutron
c.different energy states
d.different half-lives
e.different atomic number

16.True regarding isomeric transition

a. ^{99}Mo decays by the emission of beta particle with simultaneous emission of gamma rays

b. $^{99}T_c{}^{mm}$ decay to the $^{99}T_c$ with emission of Gamma ray of energy of 140 keV

c. $^{99}T_c$ has short half-life

d. Decay of rubidium-81 to krypton -81 is an example of isomeric transition

e. isomers have different energy states and half-life

17. True regarding positive beta decay

a. one of the way of acquiring stability of radionuclide with a neutron deficit

b. a proton within nucleus changes into a neutron and a positive electron

c. positive beta particle (positron) ejected from the nucleus with high energy

d. mass and charge conserved

e. transformation of ^{18}F to oxygen-18 is an example of

18. beta emitters is /are

a. nitregen-13

b. oxygen-15

c. strontium -89

d. xenon-133

e. yttrium -90

19. True regarding X-rays and Gamma rays

a. both are electromagnetic radiations

b. gamma rays are emitted by an atomic nucleus in an excited state

c. X-rays are the result of changes involving electrons

d. In their properties, and in their interactions with matter, X-rays are the same as gamma rays,

e. Unlike alphas and betas, gamma rays and X-rays do not have definite ranges

20. True regarding Auger electrons

a. refers to outer orbital electrons ejected by nuclear energy

b. properties similar to beta particles

c. may produce Bremsstrahlung radiation

d. may be produced during electron capture

e. positively charged

21. True regarding iodine -123

a. half life –13hrs

b. decays wholly by positive beta

c. emits 160 keV Gamma rays

d. emit 28 keV X-rays

e. emit positive beta particle

22. True regarding gamma rays.

a. gamma rays energies characteristic of the nuclide that emits gamma rays

b. Iodine -131 emits mostly 160 keV gamma rays

c. Iodine -123 emits 360 KeV gamma rays

d. ^{99}Mo and ^{99}Tc emits gamma rays only

e. gamma rays have identical properties to X- rays

23. True regarding iodine

a. internal conversion of gamma rays noted in iodine -125

b. Iodine -125 emit both photoelectrons and characteristic X-rays

c. iodine 125 emit characteristic X-rays of less than 35 keV.

d. iodine -125 more suitable for imaging

e. iodine-125 half –life is 8 days

24. True regarding collimators

a. placed in front of the crystal to restrict the direction of gamma rays entering the crystal

b. The usual form of collimator is a block of lead with an array of holes orientated perpendicular to the face of the crystal

c.The performance of the collimator is determined by the number of holes, the diameter and length of each hole and the septal thickness

d. the resolution of collimators designed for high-energy isotopes is generally poorer than that of those used for low-energy isotopes.

e. The pinhole collimator is a hollow metal cone that fits over a circular detector face, and has a single hole at its point.

25.True regarding k-electron capture

a.one of the way of acquiring stability of radionuclide with a neutron excess

b.capture an extranuclear electron from the nearest (K) shell

c.increase its number of protons relative to the number of neutrons

d.the daughter nuclide emit K-characteristic X rays

e.may emit gamma rays if daughter nuclide in excited state

26.Limitations of Gamma camera

a.limited spatial resolution

b.partial volume effect

c.attenuation correction

d.count rate limitations

e.compromized image quality of distant object

27.True regarding PET

a. contains several rings of block detectors

b. uses the coincidence detection of paired 611 keV annihilation photons from positron-emitting radionuclides

c. possible to acquire and reconstruct a tomographic image without the need for collimators

d. much poorer sensitivity but better spatial resolution than SPECT

e. PET detectors typically use crystals such as bismuth germinate (BGO), lutetium orthosilicate (LSO) and gadolinium orthosilicate (GSO).

28.True regarding beta rays.

a.the range in tissue is inversely proportional to the density of the material

b.E_{max} of beta rays is characteristic of the radionuclide

c.the average energies of beta rays is about $E_{max}/2$

d.ionise atoms of material producing the track dotted with ion pairs

e.range of a few millimeters in tissue

29.True regarding positron emitters

a.antimatter

b.very brief existence

c.the mass of each electron is equivalent to 511keV

d.two photons each of 511keV emitted as result of annihilation of positron and electron

e.basis of CT scan

30.Typical performance figures for a gamma camera

a.intrinsic spatial resolution— 3.8mm ,FWHM over useful field of view

b.system spatial resolution – 7.5mm,FWHM with resolution

collimator ,without scatter at 10 cm

c.intrinsic energy resolution—10%
,FWHM at 140 kev

d.integral uniformity –2% ,centre of field

e.system sensitivity ---160 cps MBq⁻¹,Tc-99m and a general purpose collimator

31.True regarding radioactive decay

a.a stochastic process

b.possible to predict which of unstable nuclei will disintegrate

c.emits a beta particle only

d.the quantity of radioactivity is measured by transformation rate(decay rate)

e.the decay rate refers to the number of nuclei disintegrating per second

32.True regarding particles

a.radon and radium emit alpha particles

b. Alpha particles have a very short range, typically 1 mm or less in tissue

c. Beta particles cause damage to tissue in a similar manner to alphas, but less severely

d. Beta particles ranges in tissue are a few millimeters

e.Beta emitters are routinely used to deliver therapeutic radiation doses to tumours.

33.True regarding radioactivity

a.the SI unit is the Becquerel (Bq)=1 disintegration /s

b.the natural radioactive content of the human body is about 2kBq

c.imaging dose of radioactive measured in megabecquerels (MBq)

d.the activity of radionuclide generators measured in gigabecquerels(GBq)

e.1 mCi = 37 MBq

34.True regarding radioactivity

a.measured the count rate is less than the activity

b.count rate is proportional to activity which is proportional to number or mass of radioactive atoms in the sample

c.the activity of a radioactive sample decreases by equal fractions (percentages) in equal intervals of time(exponential law)

d.the half life of a radionuclide is time taken for its activity to decay to half its original value

e.ten half-lives reduce the activity by a factor of 1000.

35.True regarding the physical half-life

a.fixed characteristic of the radionuclide

b.prediction of its value possible

c.affected by heat,pressure,

d.unaffectedv electricity or chemical reactions

e.range from fractions a second to millennia

36.True regarding radioactivity

a.the activity of radioactive sample ultimately falls to zero

b.graph of radioactivity versus time plotted on linear scales is known as exponential curve

c.on logarithmic scale radioactivity and time gives straight line

d.help in calculating the activity that must be prepared at a particular time fo use at a subsequent time

e.help in storage for sufficient time for safe disposal

37.True regarding half-life of radioactive material

a.a radionuclide (stored in a bottle) decay with physical half-life

b.radiopharmaceutical in the body decay with biological half-life

c.the effective half-life is shorter than the biological+ physical half-lives

d.the effective half-life can vary from person to person ,depending on their disease state

e.the effective half-life depend on the radiopharmaceutical used and the organ etc. involved

38.Correct matching of half – lives

a.Krypton-81m ---13s

b.Rubidium-82----1min

c.nitrogen -13---10min

d.carbon-11---20min

e.gallium-68---68min

39.correct matching of half lives

a.fluorine -18---110 min

b.technetium-99m---6hrs

c.iodine-123----13hrs

d.molybdenum-99---67hrs

e.indium-111---67hrs

40.True regarding PET

a. In 2D mode, each ring of detectors works dependently on each other

b. In 3D mode the septa are used cPET images are degraded by scatter, attenuation, random coincidences, dead time and noise

d. Spatial resolution of PET is limited by the length of the positron path (a few millimetres), noncolinearity of annihilation photons (about quarter of a degree) and the size of the detector blocks.

e. . Attenuation correction is not important for PET

41.Artefact noted in gamma

camera is/are

a. a regular pattern of dark or light spots

b. A single cold spot of similar size

c. A straight line, or lines, across the field of view

d.Star-like rays emanating from hot spots

e. Irregular lines or sharp-edged patches, a circular ring or arc

42.True regarding radioactive nucleus

a.unstable nuceus

b.emit x-ray or gamma ray

c.may emit particles

d.rate of radioactive decay of a sample is activity

e.SI unit if activity is the becquerel (Bq

43.Correct matching of half-lives

a.thallium-201---73hrs

b.gallium-67----78hrs

c.xenon-133---5days

d.iodine -131---8days

e.technetium-99---20 x 10^4 yrs

44.Desirable properties of a radionuclide for imaging

a.very short half life

b.decay to a stable daughter

c.emission of gamma rays only

d.decay by negative beta paticle

e.easily and firmly attached to the pharmaceutical at room temperature

45.True regarding desirable desirable properties of radionuclide

a. emit only gamma rays

b. emit gamma rays of energy 500-3000keV

c. emit monoenergetic gamma rays

d.low specific gravity

e.readily available at the hospital site

46.Desirable properties of

radiopharmaceutical include
a.localise quickly and largely in the target tissue of interest
b.effective half life longer than the duration of the examination
c.low toxicity
d.form unstable product both in vitro and in vivo
e.readily available and be inexpensive per patients dose

47.True regarding particles
a.radon and radium emit alpha particles
b. Alpha particles have a very short range, typically 1 mm or less in tissue
c. Beta particles cause damage to tissue in a similar manner to alphas, but less severely
d. Beta particles ranges in tissue are a few millimeters
e.Beta emitters are routinely used to deliver therapeutic radiation doses to tumours.

48.True regarding technetium-99m
a.used in 90% of radionuclide imaging
b.emit gamma ray with beta particle
c.gamma emission of 140keV energy
d.short half life of 6 hrs
e.easily collimated and easily absorbed in fairly thin crystal

49.True regarding technetium generator
a.has an exchange column of zinc beads
b.the compound of the parent ^{99}Mo remains absorbed on beads
c.sterile saline solution flows through column under high pressure
d.the technetium is washed off the column (eluted) as sodium pertechnetate
e.elution takes a few hours and leaves behind the molybdenum

50.True regarding technetium generator
a.generator is delivered in state of transient equilibrium of parent Mo-99 and daughter Tc^m-99
b.elution can be made daily
c.the generator is usually replaced with after a week
d.the old generator cannot be recycled
e.the generator cannot be eluted twice a day

51.True regarding sodium pertechnetate -99m
a.taken up by tissue due to its similarity to iodide and chloride ions
b.taken up by thyroid but not fully metabolized
c.taken up by gastric mucosa ,so help in localization of Meckel's diverticulum
d.taken up by the salivary gland
e.blocked from the thyroid by administration of potassium perchlorate

52.True regarding technetium compounds
a.MDP ---bone imaging
b.HMPAO---cerebral imaging
c.DMSA ---renal studies
d.HIDA ---biliary studies
e.MAG 3 –biliary studies

53.True regarding technetium linked to human serum albumin (HAS)
a.HSA colloidal particles

(0.5micrometer) are phagocytosed in reticuloendothelial cells

b.HSA macroaggregates (15 to 100 microspheres) used in lung perfusion imaging

c.HSA colloidal particles are used in imaging of liver ,spleen and red bone marrow

d.HSA macroaggregates temporarily block a fraction of the pulmonary capillaries

e. HSA colloidal particles are used in testicular imaging

54.True regarding isotopes
a.same number of protons

b.same position in the periodic table

c.same chemical and metabolic properties

d.same number of neutrons

e.same density and other physical properties

55.True regarding Technetium labelled compounds
a.DTPA aerosol (5micrometer) --- cerebral blood flow

b.autologous cells for cardiac imaging

c.heat-damaged autologous red cells for imaging the spleen

d.sestamibi for cardiac perfusion studies

e.tetrofosmin for bone imaging

56.True regarding ^{123} I
a.more expensive than Iodine-131 and iodine-125

b.produced by reactor

c.half –life of 3 hrs

d.decays by isomeric transition

e.emit gamma ray of 159 keV

57.True regarding ^{125} I
a.long half life of 13 days

b.emit low photon energy gamma ray(around 130 keV)

c.may be labeled with hippuran for renal studies

d.more expensive than ^{123} I

e.used for brachytherapy

58.True regarding SPECT
a.multiple views must be obtained at precisely known angles

b.the centre of rotation of camera must not move during data collection

c.the face of camera must remain accuratelt parallel to the long axis of the patients

d.camera non- uniformities appear as ring artefact in reconstruction

e.the mechanical and electronic axes of the camera must not be accurately aligned

59.True regarding Iodine
a.iodine-131 is used for thyroid ablation

b.iodine -125 is used as brachytherapy seeds

c.iodine -123 is used for imaging

d.iodine -131 is used for imaging

e.iodine 123 is produced by electron capture

60.True regarding Xenon-133
a.produced in a cyclotron

b.half-life of 5.2 days

c.emits beta rays only

d.inert gas

e.used in lung ventilation imaging

61.True regarding Krypton-81m
a.inert gas

b.half life of 13s

c.emits 190 keV gamma rays

d.generator produced

e. ^{81}Rb serves as parent

62.True regarding Krypton -81m
a.the generator producing ^{81}Kr^m is eluted with normal saline

b.pure ^{81}Kr^m is used in pulmonary

ventilation studies

c.parent ^{81}Rb has short half life (4.7 hr)

d. parent ^{81}Rb must be used on the day of delivery

e. ^{81}Kr^m emits gamma ray

63.True regarding technetium generator

a.the daughter and parent decay together with a half life of the parent ,67 hrs

b.the eluents decays with its own half-life of 6hrs

c.the strength of successive eluents diminishes in line with the decay of ^{99}Mo

d.elution takes a few minutes

e.elution can be made daily

64.True regading radionuclide

a. breast uptake of ^{67}Ga-gallium citrate is normal

b. uptake of ^{18}F-FDG in brown fat within the neck and superior mediastinum is normal

c. Beta-emitting radionuclides are most commonly used for therapy

d. measurement of glomerular filtration rate (GFR) is done with with chromium-51 (^{51}Cr) EDTA

eThe urinary excretion of cyanocobalamin labelled with cobalt-57 is used to diagnose vitamin B$_{12}$ malabsorption (Schilling's test).

65.True regarding use of radionuclide

a. ^{111}In DTPA (intrathecal)---CSF study

b. ^{99m}Tc HMPAO----blood brain barrier study

c. ^{99m}Tc HMPAO----ictal SPECT

d. ^{18}F fluorodeoxyglucose---interictal PET

e. ^{123}I sodium iodide-----thyroid scintigraphy

66.True regarding indium

a.^{111}I cyclotron produced while I-113m is generator produced

b. ^{111}I decays by electron capture

c. ^{111}I has half –life of 67 hrs while I-113m has half-life of 100 min

d. ^{111}I emit 173 and 247 keV while I-113m emit gamma rays of 300 keV

e. ^{111}I is used to label white blood cells and platelets for locating abscesses and thromboses,respectively

67.True regarding use of radionuclide

a. ^{99m}Tc nanocolloid—Lymphoscintigraphy

b. ^{99m}Tc red blood cells--Cardiac ventriculography (gated study)

c.^{18}F fluorodeoxyglucose---Myocardial viability study

d. ^{99m}Tc red blood cells---congenital shunt study

e. ^{99m}Tc phosphines----Myocardial perfusion scan

68.True regarding Thallium-201

a.generator produced

b.half-life of 73 hrs

c.decays by electron capture

d.emit 80 keV X-rays

e.thallous chloride is used in myocardial perfusion

69.True regarding disposal of radioactive waste

a.containment and decay

b.dilution by dispersal to the environment

c.^{133}Xe and ^{99}Tc^m should be exhausted to the exterior of the building

d.exhaust to exterior desirable but

not necessary in case of $^{88}Kr^m$
e. aqueous liquid waste diluted with water and disposed off via designated sinks or sleuce

70. Myocardial perfusion scan uses

a. ^{201}Tl (thallous chloride)--- K+ analogue indicating perfusion (ischaemic heart disease) (delayed uptake reflects viability)
b. ^{99m}Tc isonitriles---Cationic complexes taken up by myocytes in proportion to blood flow
c. ^{99m}Tc teboroxime---Lipophilic compound which accumulates by diffusion
d. ^{99m}Tc phosphines----Uptake proportional to blood flow
e. ^{99m}Tc red blood cells---Blood pool label

71. Radionuclide produced by generator is /are

a. technetium-99m
b. Krypton-81m
c. indium-113m
d. rubidium-82
e. iodine-123

72. True regarding SPECT

a. provide map of the concentration of radionuclide in the organ of interest
b. limitations of SPECT are collection efficiency of gamma rays, attenuation of gamma rays and limited time of collection
c. less stringent demands on the design and performance of gamma cameras than conventional imaging
d. resolution of SPECT is superior to that of conventional gamma camera but inferior to CT
e. resolution increases with the radius of rotation of the camera

73. The radionuclide produced by reactor is /are

a. iodine -131
b. xenon-133
c. molybdenum-99
d. technetium-99m
e. Krypton-81m

74. The radionuclide produced in cyclotron is /are

a. fluorine -18 and technetium-94m
b. iodine -123
c. gallium-67
d. indium-111
e. thallium-201

75. Positron emitters is /are

a. fluorine-18 (half life -110min)
b. carbon-11 (half life -20min)
c. notrogen-13 (half life -10min)
d. oxygen -15 (half life -2min)
e. rubidium-82 (half life -75s)

76. True regarding use of radionuclides

a. Alveolar permeability study---^{99m}Tc DPTA aerosol
b. Oesophageal transit and reflux---^{99m}Tc sulphur colloid
c. GI bleed study--^{99m}Tc sulphur colloid and ^{99m}Tc labelled red cells
d. Meckel's diverticulum scintigraphy---^{99m}Tc pertechnetate
e. White cell scintigraphy---^{99m}Tc leucocytes

77. True regarding uses of radionuclide

a. cholecystitis and biliary dyskinesia---^{99m}Tc iminodiacetic acid derivatives
b. pyrexia of unknown origin-----^{67}Ga gallium citrate
c. Splenic scintigraphy----Heat damaged ^{99m}Tc labelled red blood cells
d. Gastric emptying

study(Dumping)---^{111}In DTPA in orange juice (liquid phase
e. Vomiting (gastroparesis)--- ^{99m}Tc sulphur colloid in egg (solid phase)

78. Ventilation –perfusion scan uses

a. ^{123}I fatty acids
b. ^{99m}Tc albumin Macroaggregates
c. ^{99m}Tc aerosols
d. ^{133}Xe gas
e. ^{81m}Kr gas

79. True regarding positron emitter

a. fluorine -18 is most commonly used in the form of 2-FDG
b. strontium-82 generator is used to produce rubidium-82
c. rubidium-82 can be used for myocardial perfusion imaging
d. technetium-94m is produced in cyclotron
e. technetium half –life is 50 min

80. True regarding preparations of radiopharmaceuticals

a. simple mixing of the radionuclide with the compound to be labeled
b. use of shielded syringes to transfer the components between sterile vials
c. use of glove box or a sterile laminar down-flow cabinet
d. cabinet located in the room that is under a positive pressure of filtered sterile air
e. all surfaces impervious

81. True regarding quality control of radionuclide

a. 6mm lead is used to block gamma rays of ^{99}Tc^m to test contamination with ^{99}Mo
b. cromatography for testing for free pertechnetate in a labeled ^{99}Tc^m
c. spot color test for alumina

detection
d. sterility testing
e. pyrogen testing

82. True regarding planar imaging

a. radiopharmaceutical usually given by oral route
b. the most commonly used radionuclide is technetium -94m
c. gamma rays can be focused
d. multihole collimator is used to delineate the image from the patients
e. the gamma camera has heavy lead shielding

83. True regarding multihole collimator

a. a molybdenum disc typically 25mm thick and upto 400 mm in diameter
b. has some 20000 closely packed circular or hexagonal holes, each about 2.5 mm in diameter
c. holes seprated by 0.3 mm thick septa
d. the half value layer of lead for ^{99}Tc gamma rays is 0.3 mm
e. each hole only accepts gamma rays from a narrow channel

84. True regarding crystal used in gamma imaging

a. usually made of potassium iodide(9-12 mm thick)
b. crystal activated with a trace of thullium
c. hygroscopic
d. damaged by temperature change
e encapsulated in an aluminium cylinder with one transparent face

85. True regading PET

a. the point of origin ,not line of origin of gamma rays resulting of annihilation is important b.coincidence detection eliminates stray and scattered radiation

c.conventional lead collimators are needed to eliminate scattered radiation

d.the toatal path travelled by the two gamma rays in the attenuating medium is always equal to the thickness of the patients in that projection

e.coincident detection of the attenuation correction is e^{muL} for all coincident events arising along that projection

86. True regarding gamma imaging

a.absorbs 90% of ^{99}Tc^m gamma rays

b.absorbs 30% of ^{131}I gamma rays

c.produce some 5000 light photons in response to each gamma photon

d.light photons travels in all direction

e.light lasts less than a microsecond

87.True regarding crystal used in gamma imaging

a.coated with reflecting titanium compound

b.a light guide maximize transfer of light from the crystal to the photomultiplier

c.crystal is fragile

d.made of usually sodium iodide

e.hygroscopic

88.Beta emitters is/are

a.carbon-11

b.carbon-14

c. Cobalt-58

d.fluorine -18

e.iodine -131

89.True about photomultipliers used in gamma camera

a.evacuated glass envelope

b.has photocathode that absorb and emit photoelectron

c.has a series of dynodes connected to progressively increasing negative potentials

d.dynodes emit light

e.the amplification factor is very sensitive to changes in the overall voltage (about 1 KV)

90.True regarding collimator used in gamma camera

a.convergent collimator reduces FOV and magnifies the image

b.convergent collimator useful in imaging of children/small organs

c.a pinhole collimator produce a magnified but inverted image

d.divegent and convergent collimator suffer from geometrical distortion

e.FOV and in-air sensitivity both vary with distance in divegent and convergent collimator

91.True regarding pulse height spectrum.

a.only pulses in the photopeak are of use in locating the position of the radioactivity in the patients

b.PHA is used to reject the pulses in tail

c.photopeak comprises pulses produced by the Compton interaction

d.photopeak doesnot vary in peak

e.tail comprises pulses of lower energy produced by photoelectric interaction

92.True regarding pulse height analyser

a.The X-pulses enter a PHA

b.PHA reject pulses that are lower/higher than a preset value

c.PHA select those pulses(counts) that lie outside window of the photopeak

d.The window is set at 126-154 keV ,centered at 140 keV in case of $^{99}Tc^m$

e.two or three windows is used simultaneously in case of ^{67}Ga or ^{111}In

93.True regarding gamma camera

a. the 400 mm camera is used for general purpose

b. mobile camera for cardiac imaging has 650mm of field

c. mobile camera for cardiac imaging has 15mm thick crystal

d. camera for bone and gallium imaging has a large field of of 500mm

e.intensive care units use general purpose gamma camera

94.True regarding collimators used in gamma camera

a.collimator the most commonly used with a 400mm camera is convergent hole collimator

b.the FOV and in-air sensitivity are the same at all distances in parallel hole collimator

c.divergent hole collimator enables larger FOV with a smaller-diameter camera

d.divergent hole collimator magnifies the image

e.divergent hole collimator allows large organ such as lung to be imaged

95.True regarding the sensitivity of a collimator of gamma camera

a.refers to the proportion of gamma rays falling on collimator from one directions that pass trough the holes

b.typical value more than 1%

c.the more holes in the collimator the greater the sensitivity

d.the norrower holes in the collimator ,the greater the sensitivity

e.the shorter holes in the collimator, the greater the sensitivity

96.True regarding uses of radionuclide

a. Hypertension (renovascular disease)---- Captopril renography(^{99m}Tc MAG3)

b. Renal tract obstruction------ Diuresis renography(^{99m}Tc DTPA)

c. Renal scarring-----Static renal scintigraphy(^{99m}Tc DMSA)

d. Vesicoureteric reflux---Indirect micturating cystogram(^{99m}Tc MAG3)

e. Adrenal medullary tumour----^{123}I MIBG

97.True regarding ^{123}I

a.more expensive than Iodine-131 and iodine-125

b.produced by reactor

c.half –life of 3 hrs

d.decays by isomeric transition

e.emit gamma ray of 159 keV

98.True regarding spatial resolution of gamma camera

a.resolution is best close to the collimator

b.the wider the hole ,the better the resolution

c.the shorter the hole ,the better the resolution

d.the better the resolution ,the less the sensitivity

e.at the cost of FOV ,reolution and sensitivity both can be maximized

99.Desirable properties of a radionuclide for imaging

a.very short half life

b.decay to a stable daughter

c.emission of gamma rays only

d.decay by negative beta paticle

e.easily and firmly attached to the pharmaceutical at room temperature

100.True regarding uses of radionuclide

a.SOL in the brain and sarcoma----- tumour staging(thallous chloride)

b.thyroid cancer –whole body scintigraphy(^{131}I sodium iodide)

c. Skeletal metastases---bone scintiraphy (^{99m}Tc polyphosphate)

d.tumour response and tumour recurrence(^{18}F fluorodeoxyglucose)

e.insulinoma and carcinoid tumour - --Somatostatin receptor study(^{111}In pentetreotide)

101.True regarding collimators of gamma camera

a.high reolution collimators have more and smaller holes and lower sensitivity

b.high-sensitivity collimator has fewer and larger holes and poorer resolution

c.high resolution collimators is used for dynamic imaging

d.low energy collimator is used with ^{99}Tc^m

e.medium energy collimators are used with ^{111}In,^{67}Ga,^{131}I

102.True regarding seprate areas for a nuclear medicine facility

a.the preparation and storage of radioactive materials

b.the injection of patients

c.patients to wait to allow uptake of the radiopharmaceuticals into the organ of interest

d.imaging

e.temporary storage of radioactive wastes

103.limiting factor for imaging time in nuclear imaging is /are

a.the ability of the patients to remain still

b.the biological removal of the radioactivity from the organ of interest

c.the workload required for the camera

d.the need for multi imaging for dynamic studies such as cardic imaging

e.noise level

104.uses of radionuclide calibrators is/are

a.determination of radiopharmaceutical activities after delivery by the manufacturer

b.dosage of solution for injection and oral application

c.checking elute activities from generators (like Tc -99m,In-113m

d.measurement of residual activities after injections

e.determination of attenuation of different materials (glass ,plastic containers)

105.True regarding Dynamic imaging

a.helps in study of the function of kidneys ,lungs ,the heart

b.renogram is done using iodine - 123-labelled hippuran

c.in MUGA cardiac study ,seprate images ,each lasting 40ms,are acquired at 20-30 different points in each cardiac cycle

d.at each points ,several hundred successive images are added ,pixel by pixel ,to improve statistics and so reduce noise.

e.quantitative data about heart function can be extracted from

MUGA study

106. True regarding uses of radionuclides
a. Neuroblastoma--^{123}I MIBG
b. Tumour hypoxia---Hypoxia imaging(^{18}F fluoromisonidazole)
c. Sentinel node detection— Lymphoscintigraphy(^{99m}Tc nanocolloid)
d. Adrenal medullary tumour---^{123}I MIBG
e. Renal scarring---^{99m}Tc DMSA

107. True regarding SPECT
a. a gamma camera with pinhole collimator rotates in a circular orbit around the patients
b. every 16°, the camera halts for 20-30s and acquires a view of the patients
c. the sensitivity is improved by a dual or triple-headed camera
d. the 60 sets of data (or two-dimentional projections) are synthesized into a set of transverse images
e. there are fewer counts from the centre than the edges of the patients due to gamma ray attenuation

108. True regarding reconstruction algorithm in SPECT
a. filtered back-projection produce image free of star artefact
b. an area of very high activity (the bladder) can cause streaking artefact in filtered back-projection
c. Iterative reconstruction is more sensitive to star artefact
d. Iterative reconstruction is insensitive to noise
e. . Iterative reconstruction permit an image reconstruction with incomplete data acquisition

109. True regarding atom
a. charge of proton 1.6 x 10^{-19} coulomb
b. weight of proton 1.7 x 10^{-27} kg
c. electron weight 1/2000th the mass of the proton
d. nuclear force bind the electron to the nucleus
e. the energy levels of electrons are equally spaced

110. True regarding particles
a. radon and radium emit alpha particles
b. Alpha particles have a very short range, typically 1 mm or less in tissue
c. Beta particles cause damage to tissue in a similar manner to alphas, but less severely
d. Beta particles ranges in tissue are a few millimeters
e. Beta emitters are routinely used to deliver therapeutic radiation doses to tumours.

111. True regarding atom
a. protons provide stability in the nucleus
b. nucleons refers to the total number of protons and neutrons
c. nuclide is defined by a particular combination of atomic number and mass number
d. isotopes refers to nuclide with the same number of neutrons but different numbers of protons
e. a nuclide may be radioactive because of too many or too few neutrons

112. True regarding the SPECT
a. can be severely photon -limited
b. high noise

c.thinner slice reduce the noise
d.can be reduced by mathematical filtering
e.can be reduced by filtered back projection

113.True regarding negative beta decay
a.neutron is converted into a proton with emission of electrons
b.a nuclear process
c.unchanged mass number of the nucleus
d.charge of nucleus increases by one
e.favoured by nuclides which have too many neutrons

114.Factor that imposes constraint on maximum count rate is /are
a.the decay time of the scintillator has a time constant of 0.2microsecond
b.the camera preamplifier 's signal tailing
c.processing time of the pulse height analyser
d.processing time of pulse arithmetic circuit
e. time taken by radionuclide to reach region of interest

115.correct matching regarding effective dose
a.infection (Gallium-67 citrate ,150 MBq)—effective dose 15 mSv
b.infection (indium-111 leucocytes,20Mbq)---effective dose 7mSv
c.tumour (iodine-123 MIBG,400Mbq)---effective dose 5mSv
d.thyroid (iodine -123 iodide,20Mbq)---effective dose 4mSv
e.brain (Fluorine,18 FDG,400

MBq)---effective dose 3mSv

116.True regarding personal protection in handling radionuclides
a.keep the radionuclides bottles inside lead pots
b.keep arms behind a lead barrier during labelling and loading of syringes of radionuclides
c.syringes protected by heavy metal ,tungsten or lead glass sleeves
d.venting of syringes in air
e.use of waterproof (double latex) surgical gloves

117.True regarding PET
a.micromolar quantities of radiopharmaceutical can be used
b.$C^{15}O$ act as very good marker of RBC
c.fluorine -18 is used to study sugar metabolism
d.may be used for strictly quantitative work
e.Germanium-68 is used for attenuation correction

118.correct matching regarding effective dose
a.infection (Gallium-67 citrate ,150 MBq)—effective dose 15 mSv
b.infection (indium-111 leucocytes,20Mbq)---effective dose 7mSv
c.tumour (iodine-123 MIBG,400Mbq)---effective dose 5mSv
d.thyroid (iodine -123 iodide,20Mbq)---effective dose 4mSv
e.heart (technetium-99m MIBI,400Mbq)---effective dose 3mSv

119.True regarding PET
a.spatial resolution is about 5mm at the centre but increases with radial

resolution

b.random coincidences and scattered radiation give a high background radiation

c. tungsten interplane septa is used to as collimator

d.cyclotron is needed to be present close to the PET

e.when the bems are collimated each image is a three-dimentional silce

120.The advantage of the sodium iodide crystal ,doped with about 0.1% thallium

a.a high density and high atomic number ,so good gamma ray stopping efficiency for a given crystal thickness

b.the high atomic number favours a photoelectric interaction

c.thalliun gives high conversion efficiency of the order of 10%

d.a short dead time in crystal

e.cheap in production

121.Advantages of Tc -99m for radionuclide imaging is /are

a.a mono-enegetic gamma ray ,facilitating pulse height analysis

b.favourable the gammay ray energy 100 kev

c. high LET radiations emitted

d.appropriate half –life and a decay product that delivers negligible dose

e.readily available as an elute from a Mo-99/Tc-99m generator

122.Methods to deal with a radioactive spill is/are

a.clear the area of non-essential persons

b.wear gloves ,aprons and overshoes

c.mop the floor with absorbent pads

d.seal the swabs with plastic bags

e.cordon off the area or cover it with impervious sheeting

123.The quality of radionuclide images is influenced by

a.the number of counts

b.the ability of radiopharmaceutical to concentrate in the region of interest

c.the presence of, and ability to discriminate against ,scattered radiation

d. spatial and temporal linearity of the imaging device

e. uniformity and system resolution of the imaging device

124.True ragarding personal ptrotection in handling the radionuclides.

a.use of lead rubber aprons to protect against $^{99}Tc^m$

b.regular washing of hands at special hands-free designated washbasins

c.decontamination with water and detergent used when spillage

d.contaminated swabs packed in plastic bags

e.use of special detergent in case of obstinate contamination

125.Quality control of radionuclide include

a.radionuclide purity

b.radiochemical purity

c.chemical purity

d.sterility testing and pyrogen testing

e.response of the radionuclide calibrator

126.True regarding spatial resolution of SPECT

a. may be no better than 18mm

b. worse than conventional gamma

image

c. worse than X-ray CT

d. improved by high –sensitivity collimators used in SPECT

e. no effect of pixel matrix

127. True regarding neutrino

a.released during beta decay and electron capture

b.an extremely small mass

c.no charge

d.interacts extremely weekly with matter

e.no effect on patients

128. True regarding SPECT.

a.the image reconstruction process often magnifies the effect of noise

b.automatic balancing of the photomultipliers are desirable

c.an elliptical orbit may improve resolution

d.three or four camera may improve sensitivity of SPECT

e.the photomultipliers affected by the earth's magnetic field

129. True regarding radionuclides

a.Indium-111,2.8 day half-life,emit 173 keV and 247 keV gamma rays,labeling blood products

b.Iodine -123,13hr half –life, emit 160 keV gamma rays ,used for thyroid imaging

c.Iodine-131,8days half-life,emit 360 keV gamma rays and negative beta particle,used in metastases from carcinoma of thyroid

d.Gallium-67,72 hrs half-life,emit 92 keV,182keV and 300keV ,used in soft tissue malfnancy and infection

e.carbon ,20 minutes half –life, emit positron giving 511 keV gamma rays ,used for Co_2 for regional cerebral blood flow

130. True regarding positive beta particle decay

a.proton converted into a neutron with emission of positron

b.mass number of the nucleus unchanged in the process

c.charge of nucleus decreases by one

d.favoured by nuclide with too few protons

e.positron has no mass

131. True regarding gamma camera

a.a wide energy window (typically about 20%) is used

b.more than one energy window can be set

c.the patients is a major source of scattering material

d.semiconductor detector is routinely used

e.wide energy window has no problem inrelation to low energy gamma photons

132. True regarding dose to the patients

a.the calculation of internal absorbed dose uses Monte Carlo methods

b.MIRD scheme is meant for calculating organ dose

c.the dose delivered by a radionuclide examination is determined by the number of images taken

d.the organs of interest and the organs of excretion generally receive highest dose in gamma imaging

e.effective dose refers to an average dose to the body as a whole

133. True regarding radionuclide dose

a.most nuclear medicine investigations deliver an E of less

than 1 mSv

b.bone or static brain imaging deliver in doses in the region of 5mSv

c.tumour ar abcess imaging with ^{67}Ga must be routinely encouraged for accuracy

d.effective dose after Technetium-99m DTPA aerosol (80MBq) is 5 mSv

e.effective dose after thallium -201 chloride (80MBq) is 18 mSv

134.True regarding dynamic study

a.renal function assessed by 75 MBq of Tc -99m labeled MAG3

b.radionuclide injected as bolus

c.deconvulation present the result as for a single bolus of activity

e.functional image displays a feature of physiological rather than anatomical interest

135.True regarding methods of reducing patients dose

a.drink good deal of water to reduce dose

b.empty the bladder frequently to reduce dose

c.avoid conception for an appropriate period following administration of long-lived (half-life of more than 7 days) radionuclides

d.male to avoid intercourse to avoid pregnancy

e.interruption of breast feeding

136.True regarding MUGA studies of cardiac blood pool

a.the patients own blood pool are labelled with Tc -99m

b.collected data frames are gated physiologically to the signal from an ECG attached to the patients

c.left ventricle is best seen in the RAO view

d.TAC is used to calculate the change in volume of cardiac chamber

e.The most important quantity derived from the left ventricle TAC is myocardial contactlity

137.correct matching

a.bone scanning (technetium -99m diphosphonates ,600 MBq) --- effective dose 5 mSv

b .lung ventilation (Krypton-81m gas ,6000 MBq) ---effective dose 0.1 mSv

c. lung perfusion (technetium -99m HSA macroaggregates ,100 MBq) ---effective dose 1 mSv

d. kidney (technetium -99m DTPA glucose ,300 MBq) ---effective dose 2 mSv

e. kidney (technetium -99m MAG3 ,100 MBq) ---effective dose 0.7 mSv

138.True regarding positron

a. the anti-particle to an electron

b.the same mass as electron

c.equal but opposite charge to electron

d.exist while has kinetic energy

d.spontaneously combine with electron when comes to rest

139.True regarding decay

a.the charge remains unchanged in negative beta particle decay

b. the mass number remains unchanged in negative beta particle decay

c.alpha decay reduces charge by two units

d.alpha decay reduces mass number by four units

e.the mass number remains unchanged in positive beta particle decay

140.Uses of SPECT

a.thallium studies of myocardial infarction and ischemia

b.quantitative cerebral blood flow

c.detection of tumours

d.detection of bone irregularities

e.cardiac gated myocardial study

141.cyclotron produced positron emitter is/are

a.carbon-11

b.nitrogen-13

c.oxygen-15

d.fluorine-18

e.xenon-133

142.True regarding pulse arithmetic circuit of gamma camera

a.combines the light pulses from all the photomultipliers according to certain equations

b.yield three voltage pulses (X,Y,Z)

c.'height' of the Z-pulse (volts) is proportional to the square of gamma ray energy (in keV)

d.The Z-pulses vary in height

e.pulses falling outside the PHA window form the gamma image

143.True regarding ^{18}F

a.most common positron emitter used in PET

b.travels about 2mm through the patient

c.annihilated by a negative electron

d.on annihilation ,produce two photons(each of exactly 411keV)

e.photons are emitted simultaneously in and practically in same direction

144.true regarding alpha particle

a.has two neutrons

b.has two protons

c.mass number decreases by four

units in alpha decay

d.alpha decay occurs in the higher atomic number nuclides

e.alpha decay emit beta particle

145.True regarding disposal of radioactive waste

a.solid wastes placed in designated sacks

b.solid wastes disposed to authorized incinerators or waste contractors

c.keeping of used generators in a secure shielded store

d.contaminated clothing and bedding bagged and stored in secure protected area

e.venting of gaseous waste to the atmosphere

146.True regarding scintillation detectors

a.effective atomic number of bismuth germinate is 51

b.decay time of bismuth germinate is 300ns

c.typical energy resolution at 511 keV is 10%

d.decay time of gadolinium oxyorthosilicate is 60ns

e.effective atomic number of lutetium oxyorthosilicate is 75

147.True regarding dynamic study

a.renal function assessed by 75 MBq of Tc -99m labeled MAG3

b.radionuclide injected as bolus

c.deconvulation present the result as for a single bolus of activity

e.functional image displays a feature of physiological rather than anatomical interest

148.Characteristics of ideal scintillators used in PET is/are

a.high detection efficiency –to

absorb and convert 511 photons into light

b.very short scintillation decay time

c.good energy resolution

d.easy to manufacture into crystal blocks

e.readily available

149.True regarding gamma rays

a.gamma rays represent transitions between well defined energy levels in the nucleus

b.are monoenergetic

c.the same nuclide may emit gamma ray with more than one well defined energy

d.gamma rays –the radiation emitted as a result of nuclear interactions

e.wavelength of gamma rays is 10^{-9}—10^{-13} mm

150.The absorbed dose delivered to an organ by the activity within it increases in proportion to

a.the activity administerd to the patients

b.the fraction taken up by the organ

c.the effective half-life of the activity in the organ

d.the energy (keV) of beta radiation emitted in each disintegration

e.the energy (keV) of gamma radiation emitted in each disintegration

151.True regarding gamma imaging

a.the number of electrons entering the PMT per gamma ray photons interaction is small

b.about 60 ev is dissipated in the crystal for the production of each visible or ultraviolet photon

c.only about one photoelectron is produced for every 100 photons on the PMT

d.The ratio of FWHM of the photopeak spectrum to the photopeak energy is a measure of the energy resolution of the system

e.The energy resolution of the system is about 40% for a gamma camera at 140 keV

152.True regarding interaction

a.the amount of energy required to create an ion pair is about 34 keV

b.x ray and gamma difficult to stop being uncharged and zero rest mass

c.the beta particle has mass and is charged ,so stopped easily (by perspex)

d.protons and alpha particles are more massive than negative beta particle and are charged(stopped by paper)

e.neutrons are more penetrating than proton ,being uncharged

153.True regarding Na(TI)

a.radiation detector used in gamma scanner

b.high stoopping efficiency of gamma rays

c.the thallium increase the light output from the scintillant

d.a long decay time ,so can be used for high counting rates

e.non hygyroscopic

154.Scintillators used in PET is/are

a.bismuth germinate

b.lutetium oxyorthosilicate

c.gadolinium oxyorthosilicate

d.sodium iodide

e.calcium zinc phosphate

155.Scintillation detectors is /are

a.caesium iodide doped with thallium

b.bismuth gremanate

c.cadmium tungstate

d.reare erth ceramic oxides

e.sodium iodide doped with thallium

156.True regarding sinogram in PET

a.the two opposite detectors measure only the sum of the activity present along a line called the line of response(LOR)

b.the summed count of each LOR is plotted as a function of its angle to and shortest distance from the centre of the scanner

c.comprises a number of blurred sine waves with different amplitudes and phases,referring to the composite intensity plot

d.each transverse slice through the patients has its own sonogram

e.each horizontal row of the sonogram corresponds to all the LORsparallel to each other at the same angle of orientation

157.True regarding the crystal in gamma camera

a.a very thin crystal reduces sensitivity

b.a very thick crystal degrades resolution

c.a camera crystal is typically 20 mm

d.12.5 mm crystal stops most of the 140 keV photons from Tc-99m

e.12.5 mm thick crystal very much suitable to higher energies gamma rays

158.True regarding the attenuation correction in the PET

a.tranmsmission scan used for attenuation correction

b.transmission scan usually made immediately before or after the emission scan

c.transmission scan is done using a long-lived radioactive source (^{68}Ge or caesium-137) located in the scanner gantry

d.the attenuation correction is relatively small at 511 keV

e.attenuation correction doesnot significantly improves the contrast and detail in the PET images

159.True regarding detectors in PET

a.detectors are commonly made in block format coupled to photomultiplier tubes

b.simultaneous (coincident) pulses are accepted and combined by the electronics

c.there are three types of coincidences that can occur in PET----true ,random and scatter

d.lead or tungsten septa between each ring of detectors reduce the random and scatter events

e.the axial FOV is given by the width of the complete set of rings

160.True regarding collimator

a.the parallel hole collimator produces most faithful reproduction of the object

b.the diverging collimator produce a magnified image

c.the pin hole collimator produce a minified and inverted image

d.the diverging collimator is required when the required field of view is bigger than the detector area

e.the pin hole collimator is useful for very small field of view

161.True regading PET

a.the main positron emitter used in PET imaging is ^{18}F

b.the sensitivity of sodium iodide crystal for the 511 keV is much higher than BGO

c.Dual- headed conventional gamma camera with integrated coincidence circuitary can act as PET scanner

d.^{68}Ga and ^{82}Rb are not useful radionuclide for PET scan due to high half-life

e.PET images gives functional and physiological information

162. True regarding the collimator

a.long wide holes produce high resolution but low sensitivity

b.resolution increases as the object is moved away from the collimator

b.sensitivity is heavily dependent on distance of object from the collimator face

c.thicker septa is needed to prevent image degradation from higher energy gamma rays

d.in fish- tail collimator ,the holes divege in one direction only

e.a cone beam collimator is a variation of converging collimator used to image the brain

163. True regarding detector response

a.the phatom to check the detector response is usually filled with cobalt -57

b.a defective photomultiplier is seen as an area of reduced counts in the image

c.a cracked crystal appear as a linear defect

d.background radiation leaks are useful to identify contamination of the gamma camera or its collimator

e.detector uniformity of a PET scanner is checked using long lived source (^{68}Ge or ^{137}Cs) mounted on the gantry

164. True regarding three dimentional mode of data acquisition in PET

a.three- dimentional mode of data acquisition use septa

b.collect data from all the rings at once

c.increases scatter fraction from 10 % to 40%

d.increases sensitivity upto 6 times in comparison to two dimentinal mode

e.data are acquired into a three-dimensional sinogram (Michelogram)

165. True regarding gamma camera

a.pulse arithmetic circuits covert the outputs from the PMTs into three signals X.Y.Z

b.X,Y gives the spatial co-ordinates of the scintillation

c.the signal Z is produced by summing all the weighted PMT signals

d.All X,Y signals are allowed to pass to the disply system

e.The Z signal refers to the energy of the event

166. True regarding gamma camera

a.mobile camera is designed primarily for cardiac work

b.fish tail collimator is used in scanning gamma camera

c.multichannel analysers allow the photons at many gamma ray energies to be collected simultaneously

d.dual headed cameras typically contain two high resolution rectangular detectors

e.Triple headed camera is used for brain work

167. True regarding testing of resolution

a. use of thin tube filled with ^{99}Tc (line spread function)

b. The FWHM is a measure of the system resolution at the face of the collimator

c. spatial resolution can be tested with a bar test pattern (made of strips of lead) for system or intrinsic measurements

d. in practice, the overall system resolution is no better than 5mm

e. spatail resolution in PET is worsened by Compton scatter of the annihilation photons in the body

168. True regarding radionuclide imaging

a. SNR depends on the square root of the total counts

b. SNR depend on the lesion /background concentration ratio

c. SNR depend on the square root of the sensitivity of the imaging device

d. SNR ratio increases as the square root of time

e. a typical photon density in radionuclide imaging is of the order of $1/mm^2$ ($10^5/mm^2$ in radiography)

169. Favourable Characteristics of radionuclide for gamma camera is /are

a. a short half-life

b. radionuclide decaying short half-life daughter nuclide

c. emit no beta particle or alpha particle

d. low 'k' factor

e. emit gamma rays of about 80 keV to 300 keV

170. True regarding spatial resolution in PET

a. worsened by Compton scatter of the annihilation photons in the body

b. overall resolution depends on the width or acceptance angle of the detectors

c. resolution worsens with increasing depth in PET

d. usually measured using point or line sources ,often of ^{68}Ge or sodium -22

e. The FWHM of point spread functions are used tp produce the transverse radial, transeverse tangential and axial resolutions.

171. True regarding a gamma camera

a. the intrinsic detection efficiency is almost 60% upto 100 keV

b. collimator sensitivity depends on the septa thickness ,thicker septa needed at higher gamma energies

c. the sensitivity of the collimator is approximately proportional to its spatial resolution

d. system sensitivity is expressed as total counts per second per megabequerel of activity

e. collimator determines the overall sensitivity

172. True regarding the energy resolution

a. the ability to seprate gamma rays of different energies

b. the better the energy resolution ,the better the rejection of scatter

c. the better the energy resolution ,the poorer the spatial resolution

d. the FWHM of the photopeak is defined as the energy resolution

e. The FWHM of the photopeak is typically 24% of the peak energy at 140 keV

173. True regarding Technetium-

99m

a.over 90% of routine investigation is performed with Tc-99m

b.short half life

c.emit near monoenergetic gamma ray at 40 keV

d.emits beta particle

e.decays to a long half-life daughter Tc-99

174.True regading an Mo-Tc generator

a.Mo-99 absorbed on the alumina $(Al_2 O_3)$

b.0.9 % saline solution is used to elute Tc-99m

c.possible to elute the the generator daily

d.generator can be replaced daily

e.Mo-99 half-life is 67 hrs

175.True regarding energy resolution

a.better for high-energy gamma photons

b.better with $^{99}Tc^m$ than ^{201}TI in conventional gamma camera

c.affected by the effective atomic number (hence stopping power)

d.affected by the crystal thickness

e.better the energy resolution ,better the spatial resolution

176.True regarding types of collimators

a.low-energy collimators---0.3 mm septa and can be used with gamma rays of upto 150 keV

b.medium –energy collimators --- 1.4mm septa and for use upto 400 keV

c.general purlose collimator has sensitivity of 150cps MBq^{-1}

d.low energy collimator is used with $^{99}Tc^m$

e.medium energy collimators are

used with $^{111}In, ^{67}Ga, ^{131}I$

177.cyclotron produced positron emitter is/are

a.carbon-11

b.nitrogen-13

c.oxygen-15

d.fluorine-18

e.xenon-133

178.True regarding temporal resolution

a.the total time for the electronics to register the output of the photomultiplier tube is known as the dead time

b.dead time includes time from light production through pulse production to count registration

c.the counting circuit does not recognize other independent pulses during dead time

d.second pulse is ignored in non-paralysable system during dead time

e.a significant proportion of the gamma photons may be missed during dead time

179.True regarding thallium -201.

a.72 hr half-life

b.decay by K –shell capture

c.emit 80 keV X-rays

d.emit Auger electrons

e.used in cardiac ischemia

180.True regarding principles of operation of the gamma camera

a.collimator is used to establish the spatial relationship

b.the incident gamma ray produce light in the crystal

c.some light goes to PMT

d.the signal from each PMT is proportional to the solid angle subtended by the PMT at the event

e.the collimator has no role in discriminating against scatter within the patients

181. True regarding thallium -201
a. 72 hr half-life
b. decay by K –shell capture
c. emit 80 keV X-rays
d. emit Auger electrons
e. used in cardiac ischemia

182. True regarding noise in nuclear imaging
a. generally high because of the inherently small signal
b. the noise –equivalent count rate is a measure of the true coincidences against the total coincidences
c. the noise –equivalent count rate is proportional to the square of the SNR in the final image
d. maximizing the noise-equivalent count rate will maximize the image noise
e. SNR is defined as the mean divided by the standard deviation of counts per pixel

183. True regarding spatial resolution in nuclear imaging
a. the ability of the system to produce distinct images of two small radioactive sources
b. intrinsic resolution refers to the camera (crystal, photomultiplier, and position logic circuit) in the presence of the collimator and patients
c. intrinsic resolution is improved by using a thicker crystal
d. smaller spaces between the collimator septa gives lower collimator resolution but lower sensitiovity
e. collimator resolution worsens with distance in air of a source from the collimator

184. Methods of reducing dead time
a. correction using measurements of count rate for the detector system as a function of activity
b. use of buffers to store the overlapping events
c. pulse pile-up rejection circuits
d. high speed electronics
e. detector with fast scintillation decay time

185. True regarding noise in nuclear imaging
a. can be reduced at the cost of increased patients dose
b. can be reduced at the cost of worsened spatial resolution
c. to detect hot spots and cold spots of about 10% against the background activity in the body needs a noise level of less than 3%
d. is generally high due to inherently small signal
e. noise is the principal factor in determining the quality of gamma images

186. True regarding radionuclide
a. Tc-99_m is not easily bound to biologically relevant molecules
b. most show very poor selectivity (<than 20%) for organ of interest
c. hydrogen, carbon, nitrogen, and oxygen have no gamma emitting isotopes
d. sould be readily available
e. should be easy to produce

187. True regarding resolution in gamma camera
a. intrinsic resolution is primarily determined by the performance of the coolimator
b. the trypical intrinsic resolution is about 3-4 mm
c. system resolution can be obtained

by imaging a narrow line source of radioactivity (Tc-99$_m$)

d.the system resolution is substantially less than the intrinsic resolution

e.the non uniformity in the image of a uniform flood source is a useful overall measure of the performance of the crystal.

188.True regarding nuclear imaging

a.amount of radioactivity administered to the patients is limited by acceptable radiation dose to a patients

b.only some 2% of radioactivity is concentrated in the organ of interest

c.gamma rays are emitted isotopically

d.gamma imaging is not noise – limited or dose-limited

e.gamma rays could be collected for any length of time without further dose to the patients

Answer

Gamma Imaging

1.abce----For Radionuclide images , biological behavior of radiopharmaceutical is important . For example, a radiopharmaceutical excreted by the kidney will evaluate renal function whilst one excreted in the bile will depict the biliary tree. (CHAPTER 7 ,Adam: Grainger)

2.abd---Gallium -67 decays by electron capture and is used to detect tumours and abscesses as it binds to protein. (page 127/ Farr)

3.ab----90% of stable carbon nuclei are carbon -12 with six neutrons ,while 1% are carbon -13 with seven neutrons .Carbon -11 and carbon -14 are unstable and radioactive .Carbon-11 has neutron deficit while carbon -14 has neutron excess. (page 121/ Farr)

4.abc---- Iodine -131 has half-life of 8 days .It emits beta rays as well as rather energetic (mainly 364 keV) gamma rays ,so it has been largely replaced for imaging by ^{123}I. (page 127/ Farr)

5.bc---- Nearly all nuclei extant are stable.The nucleus of helium atom is known as an alpha particle .An alpha paricle has two neutrons and two protons and is stable (page 121/ Farr)

6.abcde----(CHAPTER 7 ,Adam: Grainger)

7.abcde-----(CHAPTER 7 ,Adam: Grainger)

8.abcde ----(page 121/ Farr)

9.abcde-----(page 121/ Farr)

10.abc---- Radionuclides produced in nuclear reactor cannot be seprated from the original stable nuclide as they have same atomic number and so the same chemical properties.Radionuclide produced cannot be made carrier free. (page 122/ Farr)

11.ade---- Cyclotron accelerates postitively charged ion (protons,deuterons or alpha particle) and forces additinal protons into a stable nucleus ,knocking out neutron (produce neutron deficit nucleus). (page 122/ Farr)

12.abcde----(page 122/ Farr)

13.abcde----(page 122/ Farr)

14.de---- Beta decay is seen in radionuclides with a neutron excess ,neutron changes into a proton plus an electron .Electron is ejected from the nucleus with high energy.Nearly always ,the product or daughter nucleus is produced with excess energy .Usually ,it loses this immediately ,with emission of one or more gamma photons ,leaving the daughter nucleus with minimum energy ,in ground state. –(page 122/ Farr)

15.cd----- Isomers are nuclei which are indistinguishable as regards to mass number,atomic number,numbers of protons and neutrons ,and other properties. (page 122/ Farr)

16.bde----^{99}Mo decays by the emission of beta particle but there is delay of hours of emission of gamma rays. ^{99}T$_c$ has a very long half-life (200000 yrs). . ^{99}T$_c^m$ has short half life of 6hours. (page 123/ Farr)

17.abcde----(page 122/ Farr)

18.abcde-----(CHAPTER 7 ,Adam: Grainger)

19.abcde----(CHAPTER 7 ,Adam: Grainger)

20.abcd----(CHAPTER 7 ,Adam: Grainger)

21.acd---- Iodine -123 decays wholly by electron capture and emit no positive beta particle. (Page no/Farr)

22.ae----Gamma rays energies are characteristic of the nuclide that emits them. For example ,Iodine - 131 emits mostly 360 keV gamma rays while Iodine -123 emits 160 KeV gamma rays.^{99}Mo emits both beta and gamma rays while ^{99}Tc only gamma rays (page 123/ Farr)

23.abc---- Internal conversion of gamma rays is noted in iodine - 125.In internal conversion the gamma rays emitted by some nuclei donot leave the atom but are photoelectrically absorbed within its k shell.Iodine -123 is more suitable for imaging than iodine 125 because of its higher –energy photon emission and shorter half- life (13hrs). (page 123/ Farr)

24.abcde----(CHAPTER 7 ,Adam: Grainger)

25.bde---- K-electron capture is one of the way of acquiring stability of radionuclide with a neutron deficit . It capture an extranuclear electron from the nearest (K) shell and increase its number of neutrons relative to the number of protons. (page 123/ Farr)

26.abcde----(Chapter 7 ,Adam: Grainger)

27.ace----- PET uses the coincidence detection of paired 611 keV annihilation photons from positron-emitting radionuclides .PET has much higher sensitivity and better spatial resolution than SPECT. (Chapter 7 ,Adam: Grainger)

28.abde----The average energies of beta rays is about $E_{max}/3$. (page 123-24/ Farr)

29.abcde-----(page 124/ Farr)

30.abcde--(page 189/ P P Dendy)

31.ade--- Radioactive decay is a stochastic process but it is possible to predict which of unstable nuclei will disintegrate. Radioactive decay emits a beta or gamma ray or both. (page 124/ Farr)

32abcde----(CHAPTER 7 ,Adam: Grainger)

33.abcde----(page 124/ Farr)

34.abcde----(page 124/ Farr)

35.ade----The physical half-life is fixed characteristic of the radionuclide and cannot be predicted for a given radionuclide in any way and is unaffected by heat,pressure, electricity or chemical reactions. (page 124/ Farr)

36.bcde---- The activity of radioactive sample never falls to zero. (page 124/ Farr)

37.ade----Radiopharmaceutical in the body decay with effective half-life.The effective half-life is shorter than either the biological or physical half-lives.($1/t_{eff}= 1/t_{biol} +1/t_{phys}$) (page 125/ Farr)

38.abcde-----(page 123/ Farr)

39.abcde---(page 123/ Farr)

40.cd----In PET 2D mode, each ring of detectors works independently.In 3D mode the septa are removed. Attenuation correction is particularly important for PET because absorption or scatter of either of the pair of photons will result in loss of detection of the annihilation event(CHAPTER 7 ,Adam: Grainger)

41.abcde----(CHAPTER 7 ,Adam: Grainger)

42.abcde----(CHAPTER 7 ,Adam: Grainger)

43.abcde -----(page 123/ Farr)

44.bce----Desirable properties of a radionuclide for imaging include 1.a physical half-life of a few hours .If the half-life is too short ,much more activity must be prepared than is actually injected.2.emission of gamma rays (which produce the image) but no alpha or beta particle nor very low energy photons (which have a short range in tissue and deposit unnecessary dose in the patient) .Decay by isomeric transition or electron capture is therefore preferred. (page 125/ Farr)

45.ace---- Desirable properties of radionuclide include emission of gamma rays of energy 50-300keV and monoenergetic gamma rays(to eliminate scatter by energy discrimination with a pulse height analyser (PHA) and high specific gravity (high activity per unit volume).(page 125/ Farr)

46.ace----Desirable properties of radiopharmaceutical include 1.effective half life similar to the duration of the examination to reduce the dose to the patients 2.form stable product both in vitro and in vivo (page 125/ Farr)

47.abcde----(Chapter 7 ,Adam: Grainger)

48.acde---- Technetium-99m emit pure gamma ray. .(page 125/ Farr)

49.bcd---- Technetium generator has an exchange column of alumina beads.Elution takes a few minutes and leaves behind the molybdenum.(page 125/ Farr)

50.ab-----Technetium generator is usually replaced with after a week and the old generator is returned for recycling. The generator column can be eluted twice a day. (page 126/ Farr)

51.abcde---- (page 126/ Farr)

52.abcde----(page 126-27/ Farr)

53.abcd---(page 126-127/ Farr)

54.abc---- Isotopes has different number of neuton and different mass number(proton plus neutrons) and also different density and other physical properties. (page 121/ Farr)

55.bcd--- Technetium labelled compounds ,DTPA aerosol (5micrometer) is used for lung ventilation studies cerebral blood flow while tetrofosmin is used for cardiac perfusion studies. (page 126-27/ Farr)

56.ae----[123] I is produced by cyclotron, has half –life of 13hrs and decays by electron capture. (page 127/ Farr)

57.cde--- [125] I has long half life of

60 days and emit low photon energy gamma ray (around 30 keV). (page 127/ Farr)

58.abcde---(page 273/ Farr)

59.abcde----(page 127/ Farr)

60.bde----Xenon-133 is produced in a reactor and emits beta rays and low energy (81 keV) gamma rays. (page 127/ Farr)

61.abcde-----(page 127/ Farr)

62.cde--- the generator producing Krypton -81m is eluted with compressed air and so patients inhaling air--^{81}Kr^m mixture is used in pulmonary ventilation studies. (page 127/ Farr)

63.abcde----(page 127/ Farr)

64.abcde-----(Chapter 7 ,Adam: Grainger)

65.abcd--- ^{123}I sodium iodide is used in thyrotoxicosis. ^{99m} Tc pertechnetate is used in thyroid scintigraphy. -----(Chapter 7 ,Adam: Grainger)

66.abcde---- (page 127/ Farr)

67.abcde---- (Chapter **7** ,Adam: Grainger)

68.bcde---Thallium-201 cyclotron produced (page 127/ Farr)

69.abcde-----(page 144/ Farr)

70.abcd-----(Chapter 7 ,Adam: Grainger)

71.abcd----Radionuclide produced by generator are technetium-99m,Krypton-81m and indium-113m. (page 127/ Farr)

72.ab----In SPECT , there are more stringent demands on the design and performance of gamma cameras than conventional imaging .Resolution of SPECT is inferior to that of conventional gamma camera and much inferior to CT.Resolution of SPECT decreases with the radius of rotation of the camera. –(page 272-73/ Dendy)

73.abc---The radionuclide produced by reactor are iodine -131,xenon-133 ,molybdenum-99(page 127/ Farr)

74.abcde ----(page 127/ Farr)

75.abcde----(page 127/ Farr)

76.abcde-----(Chapter 7 ,Adam: Grainger)

77.abcde-----(Chapter 7 ,Adam: Grainger)

78.abcde-----(Chapter 7 ,Adam: Grainger)

79.abcde -----(page 127/ Farr)

80.abcde -----(page 127Farr)

81.abcde----(page 127-28/ Farr)

82.de-----In planar imaging ,radiopharmaceutical usually given by intravenous route.The most commonly used radionuclide is technetium -99m which emits gamma rays of 140 keV(page 128/ Farr)

83.bcde----Multihole collimator consists of a molybdenum disc typically 25mm thick and upto 400 mm in diameter. (page 128/ Farr)

84.cde ----Crystal used in gamma imaging is usually made of sodium iodide(9-12 mm thick) and is activated with a trace of thallium. (page 128/ Farr)

85.bde----In PET,line of origin ,not the point of origin of gamma rays resulting of annihilation is important.Coincidence detection eliminates stray and scattered radiation ,so conventional lead collimators are not needed to eliminate scattered radiation. (page 274/ Farr)

86. **abcde**---- (page 128/ Farr)

87.**abcde**----(page 128/ Farr)

88..**abcde**-----(7 ,Adam: Grainger)

89.**abe**---- Photomultipliers used in gamma camera has a series of dynodes connected to progressively increasing positive potentials.Dynodes absorb electrons and emit electrons .When each electrons strikes a dynode,it knocks out some three of four electrons. (page 129/ Farr)

90.**abcde**----A pinhole collimator is useful for imaging of a superficial small organ such as the thyroid. (page 131/ Farr)

91.**ab**----In pulse height spectrum, photopeak comprises pulses produced by the complete photoelectric absorption .Photopeak vary in peak .The spread of energies in photopeak is caused by statistical fluctuations in both the number of light photons and number of electrons. (page 130/ Farr)

92.**bde**----The Z-pulses enter a PHA which select those pulses(counts) that lie within a window of the photopeak. (page 130/ Farr)

93.**ad**---- mobile camera for cardiac imaging has 250mm of field and 5 mm crystal .Intensive care units use gamma camera for cardiac imaging ,being easy to position. (page 131/ Farr)

94.**bce**-----Collimator the most commonly used with a 400mm camera is parallel hole collimator.Divergent hole collimator mminifies the image .Divergent hole collimator allows large organ such as lung to be imaged.(page 131/ Farr)

95.**ce**---The sensitivity of a collimator of gamma camera refers to the proportion of gamma rays falling on collimator from all directions that pass trough the holes .Typical value is a fraction of 1% .The wider holes in the collimator, the greater the sensitivity. (page 131/ Farr)

96.**abcde**-----(7 ,Adam: Grainger)

97.**ae**----^{123} I is produced by cyclotron, has half –life of 13hrs and decays by electron capture. (page 127/ Farr)

98.**ade**-----spatial resolution is best close to the collimator. The wider the hole ,the worse the resolution.The shorter the hole ,the worse the resolution. (page 131/ Farr)

99.**bce**----Desirable properties of a radionuclide for imaging include 1.a physical half-life of a few hours .If the half-life is too short ,much more activity must be prepared than is actually injected.2. Emission of gamma rays (which produce the image) but no alpha or beta particle nor very low energy photons (which have a short range in tissue and deposit unnecessary dose in the patient) .Decay by isomeric transition or electron capture is therefore preferred.(page 125/ Farr)

100.**abcde**----- (CHAPTER 7 ,Adam: Grainger .)

101.**abcde**----(page 132/ Farr)

102.**abcde**-----(page 132/ Farr)

103.**abcd**------ . (page 141/ Farr)

104.abcde-----(page 187/P P Dendy)

105.abcde---- (page 132/ Farr)

106.abcde-----(Chapter 7 ,Adam: Grainger)

107.cde----In SPECT ,a gamma camera with parrallel collimator rotates in a circular orbit around the patients and every 6°,the camera halts for 20-30s and acquires a view of the patients,thus 60 views are taken from different directions. (page 132/ Farr)

108.bde----Filtered back-projection produce may produce image with star artefact while Iterative reconstruction is less sensitive to star artefact. (page 133/ Farr)

109.abc---Electrostatic force binds the electron to the nucleus.The energy levels of electrons are not equally spaced.(Page 3 /Dendy)

110.abcde---- (CHAPTER 7 ,Adam: Grainger)

111.bce----Neutrons provide stability in the nucleus, so a nuclide may be radioactive because of too many or too few neutrons.Isotopes refers to nuclide with the same number of protons but different numbers of neutrons. (Page 3-4 /Dendy)

112.abd----In the SPECT,there is high noise which can be reduced by thicker slice, mathematical filtering and by iterative reconstruction.(Page 133/Farr)

113.abcde----(Page 37 /Dendy)

114.abcd-----(Page 182-84 /Dendy)

115. abcde-----(Page 143 /Farr)

116.abce----Before injection ,syringes are vented into swabs or closed containers and not into the atmosphere . (Page 143 /Farr)

117.abcde-----(Page 274 /Dendy)

118.abcde-----(Page 143 /Farr)

120.abcd---------(Page 189 /Dendy)

121.ade----Advantages of Tc -99m is favourable the gammay ray energy 140 kev,high enough not to be heavily absorbed in the patients ,hence minimizing patients dose ,but low enough to be stopped in a thin sodium iodide crystal. Tc -99m emit no high LET radiations.(Page 190 /Dendy)

122.abcde------(Page 144 /Farr)

123.abcde----- (Page 190/Dendy)

124.abcde------(Page 144 /Farr)

125.abcde------(Page 127-28 /Dendy)

126.abc----Spatial resolution is reduced by high –sensitivity collimators used in SPECT and also limited by pixel matrix -----(Page 133 /Farr)

127.abcde----(Chapter 7 ,Adam: Grainger)

128.abcde--------(Page 133 /Farrr)

129.abcde---- -----(Page176 /Dendy)

130.abc---- Positive beta particle decay is favoured by nuclide with too many protons. -----(Page 7/Dendy)

131.abc-----In gamma camera ,semiconductor detector is not routinely used .Wide energy window permits some gamma photons that have been Compton-scattered through quite large angles and may be accepted by the pulse height analyser. (Page 180 /Dendy)

132.abde----The dose delivered by a radionuclide examination is unaffected by the number of images taken-----(Page 141-42 /Farr)

133.bde-----Most nuclear medicine investigations deliver an E of less than 5 mSv.Tumour ar abcess imaging with ^{67}Ga must be not be routinely as it deliver high dose to patients (15 mSv) -----(Page 142/Farr)

134.abcde--------(Page 182-184 /Dendy)

135.abcde---------(Page 142 /Farr)

136.abd-----Left ventricle is best seen in the LAO view.The most important quantity derived from the left ventricle TAC is the ejection fraction. -----(Page 182-84 /Dendy)

137.abcde------(Page 143 /Farr)

138.abcde------(Page 7 /Dendy)

139.bcde-------(Page 7 /Dendy)

140.abcde-----(Page 134 / Dendy)

141.abcd----Xenon-133 is generator produced and has half –life of 5.3 day ,emit 81keV gamma rays and negative beta particle a,used in lung ventilation studies. (Page 176/Dendy)

142.abd-----'Height' of the Z-pulse (volts) is proportional to the gamma ray energy (in keV) absorbed by the crystal .The Z-pulses falling inside the PHA window form the gamma image. (Page 129 /Farr)

143.abc----positron emitted by ^{18}F travels about 2mm befor being annihilated by a negative electron .On annihilation ,produce two photons(each of exactly 511keV) which are emitted simultaneously and practically in opposite direction.

144.abcd---(Page 3,Dendy)

145.abcde----(Page 144 /Farr)

146.bd----Effective atomic number of bismuth germinate, lutetium oxyorthosilicate, gadolinium oxyorthosilicate,sodium iodide is 75,66,59,51 respectively. Decay time of bismuth germinate, lutetium oxyorthosilicate, gadolinium oxyorthosilicate,sodium iodide is 300,40,60,230 ns respectively. Typical energy resolution at 511 keV of bismuth germinate, lutetium oxyorthosilicate, gadolinium oxyorthosilicate,sodium iodide is 25%,25%,15%,10% respectively.-(Page 135/Farr)

147.abcde---(Page 182-84/Dendy)

148.abcde------(Page 134 /Farr)

149.abcde-----------(Page 3 /Dendy)

150.abcde----

151.ad----In gamma camera, the number of electrons entering the PMT per gamma ray photons interaction is small because about 30 ev is dissipated in the crystal for the production of each visible or ultraviolet photon and only about one photoelectron is produced for every 10 photons on the PMT.The energy resolution of the system is about 10% for a gamma camera at 140 keV. (Page 79/Dendy)

152.abcde-----(Page 12/Densy)

153.abc----- Na(TI) has a short decay time ,so can be used for high counting rates It is gygroscopic so placed in hermetically sealed container. (Page 164-165/Dendy)

154.abc-----(Page 134 /Farr)

155.abcde----(Page 164-165/Dendy)

156.abcde----(Page 135-36 /Dendy)

157.abd----Crystal in gamma camera is typically 12 mm.12.5 mm crystal stops most of the 140 keV photons from Tc-99m but is less well suitable to higher energies gamma rays.-(Page 167 /Dendy)

158.abc---- The attenuation correction in the PET is relatively large at 511 keV so attenuation correction significantly improves the contrast and detail in the PET images. -----(Page 136 /Dendy)

159.abcde--------(Page 134 /Dendy)

160.ade----The diverging collimator produce a minified image.The pin hole collimator produce a enlarged and inverted image. -----(Page 168/Dendy)

161.ace-----The sensitivity of sodium iodide crystal for the 511 keV is much lower than BGO.^{68}Ga(68minutes) and ^{82}Rb (1 minutes) are useful radionuclide for PET scan. -----(Page 136-37 /Dendy)

162.cde----long narrow holes produce high resolution but low sensitivity,resolution decreases as the object is moved away from the collimator,sensitivity is relatively independent of distance from the collimator face. (Page 169 /Dendy)

163.abcde---(Page 136-37/Dendy)

164.abcde---(Page 136/Dendy)

165.abe-----The energy signal Z is produced by summing all the unweighted PMT signals X,Y signals are allowed to pass to the disply system only when the Z signal falls within the pre-selected energy window. (Page 170 /Dendy)

166.abcde---(Page 170 /Dendy)

167.abcde----(Page 139 /Dendy)

168.abcde----(Page 173/Dendy)

169.ace----Favourable Characteristics of radionuclide for gamma camera are radionuclide decaying to a non-radionuclide or very long half-life daughter nuclide.If both parent and daughter are radioactive ,the ratio of their activities is the inverse ratio of their half-lives.The radionuclide should have 'k' factor(emitting large number of gamma rays). (Page 175/Dendy)

170.abde---Resolution worsens with increasing depth in SPECT ,not in PET.

171.bde---A gamma camera the intrinsic detection efficiency is almost 100 % upto 100 keV .The sensitivity of the collimator is approximately proportional to the square of its spatial resolution. (Page 139 /Dendy)

172.abd---True regarding the energy resolution the better the energy resolution ,the better the spatial resolution.The FWHM of the photopeak is defined as the energy resolution and typically 12% of the peak energy at 140 keV. -----(Page 140/Farr)

173.abe----Technetium-99m emit near monoenergetic gamma ray at 140 keV and emits no particulate radiation (Page 175 /Dendy)

174.abcde-----(Page 175 /Dendy)

175.abcde-----(Page 140/Farr)

176.abcde--------(Page 131-32/Dendy)

177.abcd----Xenon-133 is generator produced and has half –life of 5.3 day ,emit 81keV gamma rays and negative beta particle a,used in lung ventilation studies.
(Page 176/Farr)

178.abce----The total time for the electronics to register the output of the photomultiplier tube is known as the dead time.Second pulse is ignored in non-paralysable system during dead time.IN paralysable system the two pulses will be added.
(Page 140 /Dendy)

179.abcde----(Page 176 /Dendy)

180.abcde-----(Page 166/Dendy)

181.abcde-----(Page 176/Dendy)

182.abd----The noise –equivalent count rate is proportional to the SNR in the final image.SNR is defined as the mean divided by the standard deviation. (Page 140/Dendy)

183.ae----Intrinsic resolution refers to the camera (crystal,photomultiplier,and position logic circuit) in the absence of the collimator and patients .Intrinsic resolution is improved by using a thinner crystal .Smaller spaces between the collimator septa gives better collimator resolution but lower sensitiovity .(Page 138/Dendy)

184.abcde---- -----(Page 140 /Farr)

185.abcde---------(Page 141 /Farr)

186.abcde--------(Page 176 /Farr)

187.bc-----Intrinsic resolution is primarily determined by the performance of the scintillation detector crystal.the system resolution is substantially greater than the intrinsic resolution.The non uniformity in the image of a uniform flood source is a useful overall measure of the performance of the camera. -(Page 177-788 /Farr)

188.ace---only some 20% of radioactivity is concentrated in the organ of interest.Gamma imaging is said to be noise –limited or dose-limited-----(Page 11 /Farr)

CHAPTER 9
Magnetic Resonance Imaging

1)True statement about Magnetization vector

a)Magnetization vector is obtained by adding up of MDM of all nuclei of a sample

b) The excess nuclei in the higher energy state give a net MDM component along the field

c) For all nuclei, perpendicular components of MDM for both spin-up and spin-down add up to zero

d) Magnetization vector has spin angular momentum

e) Magnetization vector ,being parallel to the magnetic field, it can precess about magnetic field

2) True about proton density weighted images are

a)Long TR and short TE

b) As short as possible TE (15ms) is used to reduce the effect of T1

c) Long TR (1000-3000ms) is used to reduce effect of T2 on contrast

d) Greater is PD, stronger is signal and brighter the pixel

e) CSF and fat appear bright

3) True about upper and lower part of k space are

a)Data from shallow encoding gradient

b) High spatial frequenc

c) better detail

d)Stronger signal

e)Both high and low frequencies

4)True about three- dimensional imaging(volume imaging)

a) A steep gradient is used to select thick slice, enough to include whole volume to be imaged

b)Frequency encoding is used along one axis

c) Phase encoding is used along two axis including slice selection direction

d) Data processing requirements are decreased

e) Motion artefacts and phase wraparound artefacts noted

5) Artifact in MRI can be reduced by

a) aliasing can be reduced by enlarging FOV or better match surface coil

b) chemical shift can be reduced by reducing frequency bandwidth

c)Motion artifact can be reduced by swapping phase and frequency

d) Magnetic susceptibility can be reduced by use of GRE sequence

e) Truncation can be reduced by reducing phase encoding

6)True regarding gradient coil are

a) the slice select gradient is switched on during the application of the RF pulse

b)Frequency encoding gradient is switched during receive of MR echo

c)Phase encoding gradient is switched between 90 and 180 degree pulse

d)Rapid switching off of gradient produce a loud bang

e)DC current is used in gradient coil

7)True regarding slice thickness and interspaces

a)increase in slice thickness, increases SNR

b)decrease in slice thickness decrease spatial resolution

c) decreases in slice thickness increase partial volume effect

d) increase in slice interspaces reduces cross talk

e) increase in slice thickness enables larger volume scanning

8) Regarding MRI, which of following is true

a)Mri uses microwaves and magnetic fields

b)Atom with odd number of proton possess nuclear magnetic resonance

c)Hydrogen has large magnetic moment

d)Hydrogen is abundant in water but low in fat

e)Hydrogen provides the best MRI signal

9) True regarding multiecho imaging

a)Allows acquisition of more than one TE echo from one slice

b) Different TE time

c) The TR are same for all images

d) The signal strength of the echo remains same with lengthening of TE time

e) images obtained from echoes with longer TE intervals will contain more noises, and so less contrast

10)True statements are

a)Phase coherence refers to the relationship among precessing transverse magnetization vectors

b) In biological tissues, except fluids, the T2 is typically five to ten times shorter than the T1

c) $T2^*$ incorporates both the tissueT1 value and the contribution from field inhomogeneities

d)$T2^*$ depend upon the magnitude and distribution of field inhogeneities as well as the size and shape of the voxel

e) $T2^*$ is due to irreversible dephasing

11)True regarding GRE

a) Unlike 2D,in 3D GRE , slices are truly contiguous and motion artefacts are reduced

b)MP-RAGE is an inversion recovery magnetization-prepared 2D GRE acquisition

c)MP-RAGE is useful in fMRI

d) TurboFLASH is a single shot GRE

e)GRE is not sensitive to hemorrhage

12) True regarding flow compensation

a) A method for reducing flow and motion artifact

b) decrease signal intensity from flowing blood and CSF

c) Suppress ghost artifacts arising

from csf

d) Used in contrast enhanced MR angiography

e) Reduce/eliminate CSF flow void sign in the aqueduct of sylvious

13)True regarding fat suppression

a)Protons in lipid is associated with denser electron cloud than that in water molecules

b)At 1.5T, hydrogen nuclei in fat molecules precess at approximately 210Hz above hydrogen nuclei in water

c)CHESS fat suppression uses binomial hard pulses

d) CHESS does not require stringent static magnetic field

e)Additional time requirement is a major drawback of CHESS fat saturation

14) True regarding artifact in EPI

a) Breathing or cardiac pulsation cause ghost artifact in single shot artifact

b)N/2 ghosts cause duplicate images of the object

c)N/2 ghosts propagate along the frequency encoding direction

d)N/2 ghosts are due to slight mismatch in timings of the odd and even echoes

e)Gradient stability may reduce N/2 ghosts

15) True regarding T1 agents

a) Increase the rate of relaxation proportional to the amount of contrast agent

b) Transverse relaxivity is less than the longitudinal relaxivity

c)Relaxivity is proportional to the number of inner-sphere water molecules

d) Relaxivities of aqua ions are proportional to the magnetic moment

e)Magnetic moment of Gd is 8 Bohr Magneton

16)True regarding CE MRA

a)Contrast (Gd) is used to shorten T2 of blood

b) vessel appears bright

c) Sensitivity to turbulence is dramatically reduced

d) In-plane saturation are eliminated

e) Intrinsically fast

17)True statements are

a)Saturation recovery is used in cardiac perfusion imaging.

b)Spatial presaturation is used to eliminate artifact from flowing blood.

c)Spatial presaturation is used to perform selective angiography.

d)Magnetization transfer preparation is used for background suppression in MR angiography.

e) Chemical shift can be used to suppress fat .

18)True regarding gradient in EPI

a)The ramp time (time from zero to maximum amplitude and vice versa) for readout gradient must be extremely short.

b) Gradient must be capable of reaching higher peak amplitudes.

c)Higher slew rate (gradient magnetic field change per unit time.)

increase susceptibility and $T2^*$ filtering effects.

d) Drawback of high slew rate is risk of neuromuscular stimulation.

e)High slew rate gives higher spatial resolution.

19)True regarding extracellular contrast agents like Gd-DTPA

a)Contain an 4-coordinate ligand binding site to Gadolinium.

b)Contain single water molecule coordination site to Gadolinium.

c)Octadentate ligand provide thermodynamic stability.

d)Octadentate ligand has no role in excretion of contrast.

e)The Gd and coordinated water molecule are essential to providing contrast.

20)True regarding CE MRA

a)Very short TR, of the order of 5ms or less.

b)Short TE , of the order of 1ms.

c)Make gradient waveform as short as possible.

d)Elliptic centric reordering technique useful.

e)Sensitivity to saturation.

21)Hydrogen provides the best MRI signals because of

a)Single neutron

b)Large magnetic moment

c)Abundance in body

d)Abundance in water

e)Paucity in fat

22)True statements are

a)Tissue with large PD and long T2 give large signal and bright pixel

b)Tissue with long T1 give small signal and bright pixel

c)Air and cortical bone appear bright in all images

d)TR controls the amount of T1 weighting

e)TE controls the amount of T2 weighting

23) True regarding phase encoding are

a)Applied between 90 degree pulse and 180 degree pulse

b)During brief phase encoding , some of precessing dipoles and Mxy vectors speed up and some slow down

c) After phase gradient pulse is over , phase differences remain and are dependent on the position

d)With steep gradient, spins are all in phase and the signal will be maximum

e)Pixel size =FOV/number of phase encoding gradient

24) True about volume imaging

a) A method of spatial encoding

b) long scan time ,may be mitigated by GRE with short TE

c) Slice selection direction is phase encoded

d) Gaps between reformatted image and much of cross talk

e)2-D FT is used to decode the information

25) True regarding ^{31}P MRS are

a) Gyromagnetic ratio –17.2MHz at 1T

b) MR signal more than ^1H

c)MR signal has lower spatial resolution than ^1H

d) Indicator of energy metabolism

e) Different resonant frequency when bound to inorganic salt

e)To reduce imaging time, much larger pixel used

26)True regarding zipper artifact

a) A central line across the periphery of the image

b)Usually in the frequency encoding direction

c) Due to leakage of RF from transmitter to the receiver

d) Can also be produced by RF interference

e) Peripheral line across the middle of the image

27) True about RF(transmitter/ receiver) coils are

a) Tuned to the resonant frequency

b) Produce magnetic field parallel to main magnetic field

c)Coil should be as close as possible to the part being examined

d)Body coil is usually a permanent part of the scanner

e)Body coil is used for receiving signal only

28) True regarding matrix

a) Increase in matrix improves spatial resolution

b) Increase in matrix leads to larger pixel

c) Decrease in matrix decreases SNR

d)Increase in matrix increases scan time

e) Decrease in matrix decreases both spatial resolution and SNR

29) True statements are

a) All MRI signals are a measure of the value of Mz

b) The single most important advantage of MRI is excellent contrast resolution

c) Spin density is a measure of the relative concentration of protons that contribute to the detected signal

d) Relative spin density is greater in white matter than the gray matter

e)Mz determine the magnitude of Mxy

30) Mechanism of dephasing are related to

a)Inhomogeneities in the field produced by the magnet of the MRI scanner

b) Differences in magnetic susceptibility among various tissues the body

c)Chemical environment of nucleus(chemical shift)

d)Magnetic field gradient applied for spatial encoding

e) Type of sequence used

31) True regarding Turbo FLASH

a) Single shot GRE

b)Give excellent T2 contrast

c)Scan time of the order of 1 minute

d)Used in dynamic Gd-enhanced perfusion imaging of the heart,liver,kidney

e) Used to determine the proper delay time for CE-enhanced MR Angiography

32) True statements are

a)During quenching, helium gas may expand 5 to 40 times its original volume

b) The maximum SAR allowed is a function of the temperature humidity the patient environment

c)Magnetometer is used to measure the magnetic field homogeneity

d)Most imaging technique can be performed adequately within field homogeneity of 10ppm

e) The stability of magnetic field required for imaging is on the order of parts-per-billion in the 1Hz to 100 Hz frequency range

33) True regarding FLASH or Spoiled GRASS

a) Used for fast T2 weighting

b) Crusher gradient is used to dephase of all coherent x-y magnetization(gradient spoiling)

c)RF SPOILING prevent the buildup of transverse coherences

d)Crusher gradient is used after sampling the echo and before the next excitations

e)Unlike gradient spoiling, RF spoiling is effective even in the center of the magnetic field

34) True regarding artifact in EPI

a) Sensitive to susceptibility directed along phase encoding direction

b)T2* decay during the echo train causes blurring(filtering of high spatial frequencies) along the phase encoding direction

c)Fat suppression is not essential in single shot EPI to overcome chemical shift artifact

d) Chemical shift artifact is minimal in EPI

e)N/2 ghosts are due to imperfections in gradient

35)True regarding Multidentate ligand in Gd-based contrast

a) Octadentate

b) Required for safety

c) Provide high thermodynamic stability

d) Provide kinetic inertness with respect to metal loss

e) Enables contrast agent to be excreted intact

36)True regarding Gadolinium

a)Paramagnetic material

b)Reduce only T1

c) Gd^{+3} itself is non-toxic

d)Very low rate of adverse events and no nephrotoxicity as compared to iodinated contrast

e)Biological half life is approx. 90 minutes

37)Which of following are true about MRI

a)Radio wave is sent through the body

b)The patient is placed in a magnet

c) Absorbed radio waves are used for reconstruction of the image

d)Hydrogen nuclei absorb and emit radiofrequency energy

e)Mri measures hydrogen content of individual voxels

38)True statements are

a)In PDW images, grey matter appears brighter than white matter

b)In T2W images,grey matter appears brighter than white matter

c)In T1W images,grey matter appears brighter than white matter
d)In PDW images,CSF and fat appears bright
e)In T2W images,CSF appears brighter than fat

39) True statements are

a)FOV may be increased by use of more steep field gradient
b)FOV may be increased by increasing the receive bandwidth
c)Voxel width=FOV/number of components into which the frequency spectrum has been sampled
d)Imaging time =number of excitations x number of phase encoding steps x TE
e)Steeper is the slice selection gradient , the thinner the slice

40)True about parallel imaging are

a) A way to achieve high temporal and spatial resolution
b) SMASH and SENSE are totally parallel imaging techniques
c) Use of an array of RF detection coil to perform some of the frequency encoding
d) Images are obtained with fewer phase encode steps
e) Scan time reduced

41)MR active nuclides are

a)^{1}H
b)^{16}O
c)^{19}F
d)^{13}C
e)^{31}P

42) True about truncation artifact

a) Parallel striations
b) Appear at high contrast interfaces(between fat and muscle,between CSF and spinal cord)
c) More likely in the frequency encoding direction
d) Reduced by increasing the FOV
e) Reduced by increasing the matrix

43)True regarding surface coil are

a) Local receiver coil
b) Applied to part (spine,kneeetc) as close as possible
c) Receive signal effectively from a depth equal to the coil diameter
d) Pick up larger signal and larger nois
e)Larger voxel and FOV, better resolution

44)True regarding increase of FOV

a) larger area coverage
b)SNR decreases
c)Aliasing atefacts more likely
d) Decrease of SNR and less aliasing
e)Spatial resolution improves

45)True regarding T1

a)T1 is the time required for the regrowingMz vector to regain 63% of its original value
b) With short TR, tissue T1 differences are reflected in different signal strengths
c)) With long TR, tissue T1 differences have little influence on relative signal strengths
d)Tissue with a long T1 recover

174

signal strength rapidly after a 90 degree pulse

e) Tissue with a short T1 recover signal strength slowly after a 90 degree pulse

46) True statements are

a) GRE is also called Hahn echo

b)The principal cause of field inhomogeneities in clinical MRI is interaction of the magnetic field with the human body

c) Water and most of biological tissues have a small positive magnetic susceptibility

d)SE is much more sensitive than GRE to magnetic susceptibility

e)Chemical shift for hydrogen nuclei in fat is 3.5ppm more than that for hydrogen nuclei in water

47) True regarding HASTE

a)Stands for half-Fourier acquisition single shot turbo spin-echo

b) Scan time of the order of a second or less

c) Sensitive to cardiac and respiratory motion

d)Routine use in MR cholangiography

e)Blurring is concern in MR urography and cholangiography

48) True regarding resistive magnet in MRI

a)Produce lower magnetic field <0.3T

b)Cooling system used to remove large amount of heat dissipated by the resistive coils

c)Poor field stability

d)Emergency shutdown very fast

e) Low operating cost

49)True regardingTurbo FLASH

a)GRE that uses an RF preparation.

b)There are multiple,short TE and TR FLASH acquisitions

c) A single inversion pulse is applied before every line of the data (every phase encoding step)

d)Inversion pre-pulse may be spatially selective or nonselective

e)The Ernst angle is large

50)True regarding k-space

a)K-space refers to raw data(data as collected before the 2D Fourier transform) depicted as a 2D matrix of spatial frequencies

b)The center of k-space consists of data acquired during the strongest phase encoding gradients

c) The data in the center of k-space controls image detail

d)The outer part of k-space contain high spatial frequencies

e)The data in the outer part of k-space controls image contrast

51) True regarding free induction decay(FID)

a) FID refers to the signal that is measured just after an refocusing pulse.

b) FID results from

precession of the transverse magnetization.

c) Free in FID refers to freeing of RF pulse.

d) Induction refers to induction of voltage across the coil by precessing magnetization.

e) Decay refers to gradual decrease

of signal.

52)True regarding Gd contrast

a) Very hydrophobic
b) widely different relaxivities
c)Excellent safety profile
d)Can be formulated at high concentrations
e)Yields similar diagnostic information

53)Gd chelates with no protein interaction are

a)Magnevist
b)Gadoteridol
c)Gadodiamide
d)MS-325
e)B-22956

54)Which of followings are true

a)Proton spins intermittently
b)Proton acts like dipole
c)Solenoid coil of mri carry AC current
d)Random distribution of magnetic dipoles
e)Earths magnetic field is about 500micro tesla

55) True about T1 and T2 are

a)T1and T2 are mutually antagonistic and have opposite effect on image brightness
b)Generally speaking , tissues with long T1 has short T2
c)Images can be weighted for both T1 and T2
d)The signal produced by 90 degree pulse depends on the value of Mz immediately before the pulse is applied
e)The TR controls the amount of T1 weighting

56) True statements are

a)Increasing the number of excitations increase noise
b)A fast Fourier transform converts the K space distribution into an image of the patien
c)On tissue movement ,signals will be attributed to the wrong pixels in the frequency direction of k space
d)The steeper is the slice selection gradient, the thinner the slice
e)The steeper are the frequency and phase encoding gradients, the smaller the FOV

57) True regarding Dixon method for chemical shift imaging

a)Atomic electron of atoms affect resonant frequency of nearby spinning proton
b)The resonant frequency of the proton is about 3 ppm less in fat than in water
c) A water plus fat image is obtained by setting the TE they are exactly out of phase
d)A water minus fat image is obtained by slightly delaying the TE until they are exactly in phase
e)Chemical environment does not affect resonant frequency of atom

58) True regarding phased array coils are

a) Multiple receiver coils.
b) Signals are received collectively.
c)Large FOV.
d) More noise.

e) All data acquired in a single sequence.

59) True regarding coils are

a) Body coils gives large FOV.
b)Local coil decreases SNR.
c) Local coil promotes aliasing.
d) Local coils makes motion arefact less likely .
e)Phase array coil used in parallel imaging.

60) True regarding T_2^* and T2

a) T_2^* would be exactly equal to the spin-spin relaxation time,if applied field were perfectly uniform.
b)T2 star is much shorter than T2.
c) T2 star is in range of few ms,while T2 is in range of 50-350 ms.
d)T2 star is in response to inhomogeneity in the magnetic field.
e) T2 is characteristic of the material under investigation.

61) True regarding T1 and T2

a) T1 may be longer in a stronger magnetic field.
b) T1 value of fat is strongly influenced by magnetic field strength.
c) Percent decrease in Mxy depends on T1 time of the tissue and TE of the spin- echo sequence.
d)A long TE maximizes T2 difference because there is time for Mxy to decay.
e)A spin echo sequence using a long TE is T2 weighted image.

62)True regarding magnetic field gradient are

a)Magnetic field gradient refers to the situation wherein the magnetic-field strength varies with position along a specific direction.
b)At the is center ,magnetic field from the gradient coil is maximum.
c)High gradient strengths are useful to achieve short acquisition times and high spatial resolution.
d)The times required to switch the gradient on and off are called ramp up and ramp down times.
e) The slope of the ramp up or ramp down portion of a gradient waveform is called its slew rate.

63) True regarding echo planar imaging

a) Scan time as little as a tenth of a second or less.
b) limited spatial resolution.
c) Technique of choice for diffusion imaging .
d) Produce gradient –induced eddy current.
e)Marked sensitivity to artifacts from poor shim.

64)True regarding permanent magnet

a)Produce high magnetic field.
b)Homogeneity medium(approx 40ppm).
c)Magnetic field stability medium.
d)High fringe field.
e)Very large weight 10-35 tones.

65)True regarding Turbo STEAM

a) A single shot technique.
b)Two 90 degree pulses are applied TE/2 apart.
c) Use of a series of fast, low flip-angle readouts.

d) Capture magnetization stored along X-Y axis.

e) Used for fast diffusion imaging or black blood imaging of the heart.

66)True regarding k-space

a)The manner in which the various spatial frequencies are collected determines the k-space trajectory.

b)The relative speed at which k-space is covered determines the savings possible with a particular MRI technique.

c)The k-space trajectory for any sequence must span all the points to generate a complete image.

d)EPI collects the full k-space matrix in a single shot.

e)The data in the center contain high spatial frequencies.

67) Macromolecular Gd chelates are

a) Magnevist .

b)Gadoteridol.

c)Gadodiamide.

d)Gadomer-17.

e)P792.

68)True about MRI are

a)Z-axis along the length of the patient.

b)Magnetic field strength usually between 0.15 to 3T.

c)1T is about 10000 times greater than the earth's magnetic field.

d)Static magnetic field B highly uniform.

e)Patient become highly magnetized inside the coil.

69) True statements are

a)The steeper a gradient, less the power consumed by the gradient coil.

b)In frequency encoding direction , all spatial information is obtained in 10-20ms.

c) Increasing the matrix makes difference to total scan time.

d)In phase encoding direction, the spatial information is not complete until all the gradient steps have been completed.

e)Motion artefacts occurs in frequency encoding direction.

70) The effect on the MR image of the flow of blood depends on

a) velocity.

b)flow profile.

c)direction of flow relative to slice.

d)pulse sequence.

e)pulse parameter.

71) True regarding noise are

a) Noise is random variation in MR signal.

b) Noise occurs at all frequency and all time.

c) Noise appears worst in the areas of high PD and high signal.

d) Principal cause is scanner.

e) Noise reduce contrasts between tissues.

72) True regarding permanent magnet

a)Consumption of low power.

b) No need of temperature control.

c) Can be turned off in emergency.

d)High operating cost.

e)Initial costs are low.

73)True regarding FISP(Fast imaging with steady state precession)

a)Fast GRE technique.
b)Used to enhance the signal from long $T2^*$ component (such as fluid).
c) The phase of RF is not alternated on successive excitations.
d)The gradient spoiling table in is used .
e)Coherent magnetization that persists after signal sampling is realigned along z-axis and is made available for re-excitation.

74)True regarding half Fourier

a)Only positive phase-encoding steps are acquired along with the zero step and a few negative ones.
b)A mirror image copy of the positive data is created.
c)Reduce scan time exactly by 50%.
d)Used in perfusion imaging,MRA. HASTE, balanced SSFP.
e)increase in SNR and decreased sensitivity to motion.

75)Liver agents are

a)Gd-BOPTA(Gadobenate).
b)Gd-EOB-DTPA(primovist).
c)Mn-DPDP(Mangofodipir).
d)Iron oxide particles(SPIO)
e)Gd-DTPA.

76)True regarding MRS

a)^{1}H-MRS needs water suppression.
b)^{1}H-MRS uses almost exclusively gradient-based volume selection.
c)In order to receive same signal much smaller voxel is needed in MRS.
d)Spatial resolution of metabolite MRS is inherently lower than that of water MRI.
e)Electrons shield nuclei and so nuclei experience a weaker magnetic field.

77)All are true about effect of static magnetic field

a)Magnetic dipoles orient in spin up(parallel) or spin down (anti-parallel) direction.
b)Slightly more magnetic dipoles orient in spin down direction.
c)Mri depends on detecting spin up oriented magnetic dipoles.
d)Difference in spin up and spin down oriented protons are proportional to B.
e)Difference in spin up and spin down oriented protons are about three hundred out of each million protons at 1T .

78) True statements are

a)Magnetic field gradients are used to localize the MR signal.
b)Slice select gradient is applied when the RF pulse is switched off.
c) Phase encoding gradient is applied before 90 degree pulse.
d)MR signal is measured during Frequency encoding gradient .
e)Fourier transformation convert the data into the image.

.79)Following statements regarding multislice technique are true

a)Multislice technique make use of TR.
b) A succession of 90 and 180 degree RF pulses ,each of same

frequency, are used in multislice technique .

c)A series of up to 32 separate slices are excited in multislice technique.

d)Gap between slices is needed to avoid cross- talk in multislice technique.

e)Two or more successive 180 degree pulse are used.

80) True about effect of spin echo sequence on blood flow

a) Slow flowing blood (e.g. in a vein) appear bright.

b) Fast flowing blood (e.g. aorta) appear dark or void.

c)Turbulent flow usually appear bright.

d) Conventional T1 weighing with presaturation pulses produces bright blood flow.

e) Any signal from vessel indicate stagnant flow or an occlusion.

81)True regarding coils in MRI

a)Surface coil gives superior SNR as compared to body coil.

b) A whole volume coil is used to acquire a uniform signal from a large volume.

c) Larger surface coil yields better SNR.

d) Use coil with smaller filling factor to maximize the SNR from a given coil.

e)Linear coil yield better SNR than that of quadrature coil.

82) Signal in MR can be increased by

a) Increasing voxel size .

b) Increasing FOV.

c) Increasing slice thickness.

d)Increasing the number of phase-encoding steps.

e) SE sequence.

83)True regarding permanent magnet used in MRI

a) Can be shut down.

b) Give high field strength up to 1.5T.

c) Give vertical or horizontal field.

d) Used for claustrophic patient, children and obese.

e) Used in interventional procedure.

84) True about MRI machine

a) Faraday cage refers to wire mesh.

b) Faraday cage incorporated in the shim coils .

c) Faraday cage is used to screen the scanner from internal RF interference.

d) Pulse sequences are selected at the operator console.

e) Power cables can cause RF interference.

85)True about MRI

a)There are two types of rotational motion—orbital and spinning.

b) Image produced in MRI is due to precession.

c) Angular momentum depicts the linear motion of body.

d) Angular momentum is scalar in nature.

e) Rotational angular momentum = angular velocity/moment of inertia.

86) True statement are

a) The energy separation between the two spin states of a photon in 1T is only 17.59 x10^{-7}ev.

b) The gray matter and white matter

differ in water content by 1% only.

c) TI time of gray matter and white matter at 1T differ by 3.5 .

d) T1 abnormal tissue is usually longer than the T1 of normal tissue.

e)T1 is an indication of the environment in which the dipole is located.

87) True regarding inversion recovery pulse sequence

a) The 180 degree RF pulse is used to invert Mz.

b)The rate at which −Mz returns toward +Mz depends on tissue T2 time.

c)Magnitude of Mz is zero at time equals 0.49T1.

d)Quadrature detection allows the computer to distinguish between a positive Mz and a negative Mz.

e)STIR sequence allows selective suppression of a tissue signal.

88) True regarding k-space are

a) K-space refers to various frequency spatial −frequency components that make up the image.

b) The image is obtained by applying Fourier transform to k-space data.

c) A component at the center of k-space corresponds to a uniform intensity throught the image.

d) A component close to the center corresponds to a high
spatial frequency oscillation.

e)The orientation of the intensity oscillation in the image is determined by the distance of the the k-space component from the k-space axes.

89) True statements are

a)Spin density—short TR and short TE.

b)T1 weighted image—short TR and short TE.

c)T2 weighted image—Long TR and long TE.

d)T1weighted image is more commonly used to display anatomy.

e) T2 weighted image use short TR to minimize T1 tissue differences.

90)True regarding transmit phased array coils

a) Produce a current on each element.

b) Higher SNR.

c) Improved field homogeneity.

d)Reduced specific absorption at high field strength.

e) Used in parallel imaging.

91)True regarding MRI

a) Investigate chemical and physical properties at the molecular level.

b) The first imaging technique is attributable to Lauterbur.

c) Lauterbur coined the term zeugmatography.

d) Precession of proton about magnetic field is due to its spin angular momentum and a magnetic dipole moment.

e) Resonance refers to the change in energy states of the nuclei caused by absorption of non specific radio frequency radiation.

92) True about T1 relaxation

a)T1 is time for 63%of the nuclei to return to the lower energy state following a 90 degree pulse.

b) In spin lattice relaxation, threre is energy transfer from nuclei to surrounding structure (lattice).

c) T1 is a rate constant.

d)T1 can be measured directly.

e) T1 is always greater than T2.

93) Permanent magnetic materials are

a) Niobium-titanium .b)Alnico.

c)Barium ferrite($BaF_{12}O_{19}$).

d)Somarium Cobalt($SmCo_5$).

e)Neodymium-iron-boron(NdFeB).

94)True regarding Time-reversed FISP(PSIF)

a)RF echo is of primary importance in generating image contrast.

b)Only Stimulated echoes contribute to the PSIF signal.

c) Contrast is highly dependent upon flip angle.

d)Useful in rapid acquisition of fat – sensitive images.

e)Useful in rapid acquisition of fluid sensitive images.

95)True statements are

a)Keyhole imaging acquires only the high spatial frequency information.

b) Shorten scan time for CE-MRI.

c)TRICKS provides low- frame-rate 3D images.

d)TRICKS is particularly useful for carotid artery and pulmonary vessels.

e) Central to parallel imaging is alternating an encoding scheme(TSENSE) with under sampled phase-encoding.

96)True regarding Time-0f-Flight,MRA

a)Retention of background tissue signal.

b)suppression of a signal from flowing blood.

c)Reduction in longitudinal magnetization resulting from repeated RF excitations is referred as saturation.

d)Intentional saturation of stationary tissues makes them appear bright.

e)use of rapid slice selective RF pulses.

97)True regarding chemical shift

e)^{1}H-nuclei in a molecule experience different magnetic field strengths depending on their chemical environment.

b) Nucleus effectively shielded by electrons has low shielding constant.

c) Higher is the shielding constant , higher is the resonance frequency.

d) The variations of resonance frequency based on the chemical environment are called chemical shift.

e)The chemical shift is characteristic for a specific type of chemical.

98)True about MRI are

a)Longitudinal net or bulk magnetic vector Mz is produced by summation of spin up and spin down oriented protons.

b)There are about 7×10^{19} protons in cubic millimeter of water.

c) Detectable protons in cubic millimeter of water is about 3×10^{14} at 1T.

d)Earths magnetic field is about 50 micro.

e)Detectable protons refers to excess of spin up over spin down protons.

99) True statements are

a)AC is used to generate magnetic field gradient.
b)Slice select gradient is switched on during the application of the RF pulse.
c)A narrow bandwidth of RF pulse contain a large ranges of frequencies.
d)Slice selection is done by altering the central frequency of the RF pulse.
e)All protons of the body are excited by the RF pulse.

100) True regarding multiecho technique are

a)Make use of long TR.
b)Use of two or more successive 180 degree pulses following each 90 degree pulse.
c)Peak amplitudes of echo decrease with time constant T1.
d)The first echo may produce T1 weighted.
e)Successive echo produces increasingly T2 weighted image.

101) True about MR angiography

a) Bright appearance of slow flowing blood on SE echo is due to more effect of 90 degree pulse on unexcited blood than on stationary tissue.
b) Dark appearance of fast moving blood on SE echo is due to loss of coherence.
c) Dark appearance of turbulent flow on SE echo is due to loss of coherence ,and so reduced Mxy
d) In GRE scan, flowing blood and CSF usually appear dark.

e)Moving blood is recognized by increased brightness or phase change on GRE.

102) Signal can be increased by

a) Increasing voxel size.
b) Increasing TR.
c) Increasing tip angle.
d)Using GRE.
e) Higher field strength.

103)True about resistive electromagnet

a) It is a set of AC coils with copper or aluminium conductors
b) Consume some 5-10Kw of power.
c) Heating is of no concern in its operation.
d) Field strength limited to 0.5T.
e)Produce only horizontal field.

104) Effect of static magnetic field are

a)depolarization changes in flowing blood.
b) ECG changes above .3T, but return after exposure.
c) pregnant patient should not be exposed above 1T.
d)Ethics committee approval required above 5T.
e) MRI contraindicated in implanted pacemaker.

105)True regarding spin echo sequence

a) T_2^* is determined by spin-spin relaxation time and the H- field inhomogeneity.
b) The purpose of spin echo sequence is to remove the effect of the H-field inhomogeneity.

c)90 degree pulse is used to remove the H-field inhomogeneity.

d) 180 degree pulse is followed by 90 degree pulse.

e)Carr- Purcell echo sequence is related to spin echo sequence.

106)True regarding k-space

a) Data in the central region has high frequency component.

b) Data in the outer region has low frequency component.

c) Data in the central region represent the gross structure and contrast in the image.

d) An image can be reconstructed from a fraction of the full(containing equal portions of positive and negative spatial frequencies) data set.

e)The distance in k-space between adjacent data points is inversely proportional to the extent of the image(FOV).

107) True regarding phased-Array coils a

a) Formed by combining a series of small surface coils.

b)Individual coils are magnetically coupled.

c)Each coil elements is typically connected to its own receiver channel.

d) Yield same SNR over a large FOV.

e)Advantage are cheap cost and shorter reconstruction time.

108)True regarding permanent magnet

a)The permanently magnetized material is the source of magnetic flux.

b)The iron yoke and posts shape B_o.

c)The pole pieces serve as mechanical structure and flux return.

d) The heater keeps the magnet at constant temperature.

e) Usually produce vertical magnetic field.

109)True statements are

a)DESS or FADE utilizes both free induction decay gradient echo and RF echo.

b)Gradient spoiling and RF spoiling are used in FLASH.

c) FLASH and FISP both acquire the primary gradient echo.

d)FIST is used to enhance the signal from long $T2^*$component (such as fluid).

e)PSIF is useful in rapid acquisition of fluid sensitive images

110)True regarding projection reconstruction acquisitions

a) Sample k-space on radial lines that does not pass through center of k-space.

b)Radial k-space trajectories sample both the center and periphery of k-space on each echo.

c) Particularly useful in MRA.

d)No effect on motion artifact.

e)Under sampling produce low intensity radial artifact.

111)True regarding TOF

a)Blood outside the imaging slice is not affected by the slice-selective RF pulses.

b) Repeated RF saturate blood and produce bright signal.

c)The vascular signal increases with the velocity of blood flow.

e)Background tissue signal suppression must.

112)True regarding chemical shift

a) The chemical shift is indicated in ppm from a reference substance at 0 ppm.

b)The amplitude of the signal is proportional to the concentration of the metabolite.

c) Chemical shifts are field dependent. Attention

d)Under relaxed conditions, the area of the resonance line is proportional to the concentration of the substance.

e)Line width of a signal depend upon $T2^*$.

113)Regarding Larmor frequency, true statements are

a)The static field causes the spinning protons to wobble in regular manner called precession.

b)Larmor frequency refers to frequency of rotation of spin axis of proton around the direction of the magnetic field B.

c)Lf is proportional to product of square of magnetic field strength and gyromagnetic ratio.

d)Lf of hydrogen ---42.6MHz/T.

e)Rf has a very precise value (in water within +/-0.1Hz).

114) Regarding spin lattice relaxation, which has relatively small T1

a)Slow moving large molecules.

b)Small, lightweight molecules with little inertia.

c)Atoms in solids and rigid macromolecules.

d)Fat and water bound to the surface of proteins.

e)Compact bone, teeth, calculi, and metallic clip.

115)True regarding fast or turbo spin –echo are

a)Use of 90,180,180----sequence.

b)Phase encoding, each of 4-16 echoes with a different phase encoding gradient.

c) Scan time reduced.

d)Fat extremely dark on FSE T2-weighted image.

e)Muscle often darker on FSE T2-weighted image.

116)True about MR angiography

a) GRE produce bright signal to moving blood.

b) TOF and Phase contrast angiography uses GRE.

c) Contrast is required in GRE.

d) Reconstruction needed.

e) For good three dimensional(volume) angiography with high signal to noise, low velocity flow is needed.

117) Noise can reduced by

a) Decreasing the number of excitations.

b) Reducing the receiver bandwidth.

c)Reducing gap between slices.

d) Use of surface coil.

e) Three-dimensional imaging and multislice techniques.

118)True about resistive electromagnet are

a) Produce only horizontal field.

b) Insignificant fringe fields.

c) Can be switched off at will.

d) Ramp –up time is 2-3hrs.

e) Cheapest and smallest, weighing 2 tones.

119) Effects of time-varying gradient fields are

a) Peripheral nerve stimulation.

b) Involuntary muscle contraction.

c) Breathing difficulties.

d) Ventricular fibrillation.

e) Magnetophosphenes.

120) True about angular momentum

a) Maximum detectable nuclear angular momentum an electron =nuclear spin X Planck's constant/2 pi.

b) The lowest energy state of two interacting electron is when the spin angular momentum is in parallel direction.

c) The configuration of highest energy states between electron is usually called spin pairing.

d) The net spin angular momentum for a spin up and spin down pair is zero.

e) Non spin pairing of electrons results in ferromagnetic materials.

121) True about Fourier transformation

a) FID is in form of frequency versus time.

b) Fourier transformation of FID is in form of amplitude versus time .

c) Shape of FT of FID is asymmetrical.

d) The line width at half its maximum value is $2/T2^*$.

e) FT indicate spin density at each frequency.

122) Regarding SNR

a) Random variation in signal intensity is called noise.

b) Noise limits the visibility of high contrast structures.

c) Larger voxels produce more SNR.

d) Image averaging decreases SNR.

e) 128X128 matrix produce larger voxel than 265x256 matrix .

123) True statement

a) Defining line for safety purpose in mri is 10G-line.

b) A scan with humidity below 50%is likely to produce unpredictable image artifact.

c) In general, the force on the object is proportional to the product of magnetic field strength and the gradient of field strength.

d) Vitamin E is used as marker in MRI scan.

e) IM/IV glucagon is used to reduce intestinal peristalsis.

124) True regarding neodymium-iron-boron

a) Developed in Japan

b) Preferred material for permanent magnet

c) Produce higher field/volume

d) Low temperature sensitivity.

e) used in open MRI system.

125) True regarding spin echo

a) RARE expounded by Henning.

b) RARE use just one 90 degree pulse and multiple 180 degree pulse.

c) RARE images are highly T2 filtered causing severe blurring of all but long T2 component.

d) Fat appear subdued on TSE .

e) Advantage of TSE is its low SAR.

126)True regarding spiral scanning

a) Sample k-space on spiral trajectory .

b)The spiral trajectory begins at periphery of k-space.

c)Less susceptible to flow artifact than other rapid imaging technique.

d)Useful in fMRI.

e) Useful in coronary angiography.

127) True regarding TOF

a)TR much shorter than the T1 of tissue to cause effective spin saturation.

b)Distal flow is better retained with large flip angle.

c)Placing the imaging slice in the plane of the vessel(in-plane saturation) is desirable.

d)Flow compensation works by achieving phase coherence of both the stationary and moving spins at the time of the echo.

e)Large voxel is often used to better visualize small vessels.

128)True regarding chemical shift

a) Spin –spin coupling produce multiplets in spectroscopy.

b)Chemical shift dispersion refers to the range of chemical shifts covered by biological molecules.

c) The major metabolites in a ^{1}H spectrum cover a range of about 25ppm.

d) Chemical shift dispersion plays no role in volume selection and in acquit ion technique.

e)Position of resonance in a spectrum can be used to identify a compound.

129 True regarding atoms

a)Gyromagnetic ratio is a variable property of nucleus.

b)In the quantum theory, a frequency of 42.6MHz corresponds to a quantum energy of 2micro ev.

c)Ant parallel state of proton has 0.2micro eV higher energy than parallel state.

d)Stronger the magnetic field, faster is the Larmor frequency.

e)Net longitudinal magnetism ,Mz cannot be measured directly.

130) True statement regarding spin-spin relaxation (transverse) are

a)Mxy decays.

b)Energy transfer between nuclei.

c)Loss of phase coherence.

d)Much of dephasing due to field in- homogeneities due to patient factor.

e)1T2 is time for the MR signal to fall to 37% of its maximum value.

131) True regarding FSE

a)Scan time reduced.

b)Matrix size can be increased.

c) FSE compatible with respiratory. compensation technique.

d)Reduce spin –spin interaction, so fat bright on FSE T2 –weighted image.

e)Smaller voxel decrease spatial resolution.

132)True regarding perfusion imaging are

a)Measure the rate of delivery of blood to the capillary bed.

b) Measure metabolic activity.

c) Use bolus of iodinated contrast.

d)Arterial spin labeling may be

used.

e) Usually does not need EPI.

133) True about contrast

a)Magnetization transfer contrast uses off- resonant RF frequency.

b) Magnetization transfer is used to suppress the signal from protons bound to macromolecules.

c) STIR sequence is used to suppress signal from water.

d) T1weighting specifically increases contrast between normal and abnormal tissues.

e) Contrast agents enhances the inherent the contrast.

134)True about a superconducting electromagnet used in MRI

a) A DC solenoid ,about 1m in diameter.

b) Conductors made of a Niobium-titanium alloy in a copper matrix.

c) Use of liquid helium at 4K(-269 degree Celsius) for cooling.

d) Negligible resistance in conductor at 4k.

e) Produce horizontal field up to 3T.

135)True statements are

a)Nucleons refers to protons and neutrons.

b) Nucleons do not have orbital angular momentum.

c)Proton and neutrons have different angular momentum.

d) There are no energy levels for the nucleons .

e) Neutrons pairs themselves like protons.

136) True regarding voxel and SNR are

a) larger voxel gives better SNR.

b) larger voxel produce less resolution.

c) larger voxel require less scan time.

d) SNR= squire root of the number of averages.

e) price of improving SNR by averaging is longer scan time.

137)True regarding spin echo

a) Use of two RF pulses, 90 and 180 degree.

b) Two pulses are separated by time TE/4.

c)No of slices =TR/TE+factor related to the pulse sequence structure and performance constraints of the gradient.

d)Fat appears bright on T1-weighting.

e)Muscle,tendon,liver appear bright on T2- imaging.

138) True regarding quadrature coils

a) Circularly polarized coils.

b) Produce more spatially uniform flip angle from the RF pulse.

c) Reduces power deposition of up to 50%.

d) Increase SNR .

e) Increased homogeneity of the signal.

139)True regarding superconducting magnet

a)Produce broad range of magnetic field(0.5 to 10T).

b) High homogeneity (<10ppm) and high stability.

c) Large fringe field without active shield.

d)Emergency shutdown fast ,emergency quenching<1minute.
e)Need of high electrical power.

140)True regarding TSE

a) TSE employs a variable number of separately phase-encoded echoes per 90 degree excitation pulse.
b)The number of spin- echoes per excitation is called the echo train length or turbo factor.
c)T2 contrast in TSE is determined by the TE of the echoes used to encode the center of k-space.
d)TSE may give false impression of being T2 weighted.
e)TSE is highly sensitive to susceptibility effects of blood products.

141)True regarding fat suppression

a)Use of inversion recovery is effective in suppressing(or nulling) fat signal.
b)Null point of tissue is given by 0.69X T2.
c)The resonance frequency of fat is shifted from that of water by approximately 220Hz at 1.5T(3.4ppm).
d)The resonance frequency separation between fat and water signal decreases at higher magnetic field.
e)Efficiency of the saturation pulses depend on the homogeneity of main magnetic field.

142)True regarding TOF

a) Typically uses a gradient-echo sequence with a short TE and velocity compensation.
b)Bright fat signal is useful.

c)MT is particularly useful in intracranial angiography to suppress background of brain substance.
d)Pre saturation band is used to saturate the unwanted vessel upstream from the region of interest.
e)Large excitation flip angle may produce ghosting.

143)Gradient –based volume selection techniques are
a)STEAM.
b)PRESS.
c)CSI.
d)DRESS.
e)ISIS.

144) True statements regarding relaxation time of tissue in field of 1T

a)T2 has a value of so many tens of ms.
b)Fat >grey matter>white matter (T2 value).
c)After 3T2 ,only 15%of maximum signal remain.
d)Compact bone, tendon, teeth,calculi,metallic clip has very short T2.
e)Greater the proportion of free water in the tissue, shorter is T2.

145) True about inversion recovery are

a)Initial 180 degree pulse is used to minimize T1 weighting.
b)Initial 180 degree pulse inverts Mz.
c)Mz recovery passes through zero and reverse the direction after a time of .69xT1.
d)The whole cycle (180,90,180) is

repeated after TR.

e)The tissue with shorter T1 is suppressed.

146)True regarding Gd DTPA

a)Water- insoluble.

b)Cross blood-brain barrier.

c)Proton in fat more affected than that in water,

d)Water may appear as bright as fat.

e)Decrease contrast between pathological and normal tissue.

147) True about contrast agents

a)Positive contrast agent has more effect on T1 than T2.

b)Gd, Mn, Fe are negative contrast agent.

c) Mn^{+3}, has five unpaired electrons.

d) Fe^{+2} has four unpaired electrons.

e)$Dy^{+}3$ DTPA has five unpaired electrons.

148)True regarding superconducting magnet are

a)Liquid hydrogen used as cryogen.

b)Insignificant fringe field.

c) Expensive.

d) Weigh up to 80 tones.

e) Unsuitable for large or claustrophic patients.

149) True regarding time – varying gradient fields are

a)Produce vertigo, nausea.

b)Produce sensations of metallic taste.

c)No symptoms below 200T/s.

d)May affect cochlear implant, EEG monitors.

e)Serious fetal development problem.

.150)True about nuclear angular momentum

a)A proton pair with neutron.

b)Max detectable nuclear angular momentum= nuclear spin x Planks constant/2pi.

c)The nuclear spin is always multiple of ½.

d)Planck's constant=$6.6x^{-34}10$ j.sec.

e)Charged nucleus is spinning and has no angular momentum.

151)True regarding Fast SE (RARE or turboSE)

a)Scan time reduced by factor equal to the ETL.

b)Relatively shorter TR than conventional SE.

c) Repeated application of 90 degree refocusing pulses.

d) All echoes are collectively phase coded for a single image.

e)ETL typically ranges from 3 to 16 or more.

152)True regarding shimming

a)Process of maximizing the homogeneity of the static magnetic field.

b)Standard linear shimming uses the three gradient coils.

c)Higher order shimming allows to improve to a value better than 1ppm over a specified volume.

d)Higher order shimming is needed for spectroscopy ,spiral imaging and functional brain imaging.

e)Shimming is difficult to achieve in foot,neck,and bilateral breast imaging.

153)True regarding superconducting magnet

a)Exhibit zero electrical resistance

above critical temperature.

b)Background magnetic field affect the superconductivity of superconductor.

c)Type II superconductors does not maintain superconductivity in high magnetic field.

d)Type II superconductors are niobium-titanium (NbTi) and niobium-tin(NbSn).

e)Most MRI magnets use niobium-titanium.

154)Correct matching

a)RARE –Henning.

b)EPI—Mansfield.

c)GRASE—Feinberg and Oshio.

d)Hyper echoes—Henning and Scheffler.

e)Zeugmatography—Lauterbur.

155)True regarding DIXON method of nulling fat

a) The resonance frequency of fat is slightly lower than that of water protons.

b)Fat and water magnetization are in phase for echo times of 2.3msec,6.9msec etc at 1.5T.

c)In Dixon method, two acquisitions with approximately chosen echo times(in phase and out of phase) are taken.

d)Help in characterization of tissues.

e)Require perfect field homogeneity.

156)True regarding TOF

a)2D TOF is usually acquired in sequential fashion.

b)2D TOF has better spatial resolution than 3D TOF.

c)Use of 3D TOF is limited to vessel with moderately high rates of flow.

d)There is gradient of blood signal intensity in 3D TOF.

e)Gradual decrease in flip angle is used in TONE.

157)Correct matching of ¹H-MR spectroscopy

a) Alanine-- 1.48ppm.

b)NAA –2.00ppm.

c)Choline—3.50ppm.

d)Inositol(scyllo)—3.35ppm.

e)Creatine—3.00ppm.

158)Tue about Mxy and Mz are

a)Mxy is produced by tipping Mz and is due to phase coherence of dipoles.

b)Mxy is parallel to B

c)Mxy rotates in xy plane at twice the Lf.

d)Only Mxy produce MR signal, Mz does not.

E)The signal produced by 90degree pulse depends on the value of Mz immediately before pulse is produced.

159)True statements regarding spin-spin relaxation are

a)Causes of T2 dephasing are machine factor and tiny additional field(around 100microT) produced by each neighboring proton.

b)Local variation in magnetic field least in solids and rigid micomolecules.

c)Local variation in magnetic field greatest free water,amniotic fluid, and csf.

d)Fat<water<water bound to surface protein.

e)Spleen>liver,   Renal

medulla>cortex.

160) True regarding inversion recovery sequence is

a) Produce T2-weighted image.
b) Time to inversion (TI) is used as T1 contrast control.
c) TR used is about 2T1 to ensure nearly total recovery between pulses.
d) Time consuming ,especially at higher field strength.
e) Gives poor grey –white discrimination.

161) True about Gadolinium are

a) Has nine unpaired electron.
b) Strongly paramagnetic.
c) Very toxic.
d) Chelated to DTPA.
e) No contraindication in renal failure .

162) True about supra-paramagnetic contrast

a) Minute particles(30nm) of Fe_3O_4.
b) Dysprosium DTPA .
c) Produce local magnetic field gradient and shorten T2*,nd T1.
d) Areas of uptake appear bright.
e) Called bulk susceptibility or negative contrast agent.

163) True regarding superconducting electromagnet

a) Takes several minutes for the coil to cool down and the current to build.
b) Power is never removed.
c) Current continues to flow while using virtually no power.
d) Liquid gas is consumed to maintain the low temperature.
e) Some 200Kw energy remains stored within the superconducting coil.

164) True regarding acoustic noise in MR

a) With GRE,decreases with higher gradient amplitudes and higher field strength .
b) Hearing protection required to prevent irreversible damage at 90Db.
c) The machine limit acoustic noise is 140 although they do not exceed 120dB.
d) Earplugs reduce noise by 10-30dB.
e) No possibility of hearing damage to fetus.

165) True statement about MDM are

a) Magnetic dipole moment of a magnet / wire loop indicates how quickly a magnet/wire loop will align along a magnetic field.
b) Larger the electron flow , the less quickly the loop align in the magnetic field.

c) The larger area loops align faster than the smaller loops for given electron flow.
d) Electron orbiting around nucleus has magnetic dipole moment.
e) The MDM of L shell electron is equal to one Bohr Magneton.

166) True regarding superconducting magnet

a) The entire magnetic system must be maintained at about 4 degree

Celsius.

b) Dewar refers to double walled container designed to hold low temperature materials.

c) Liquid nitrogen is used.

d) Liquefied helium gas has very high boiling point.

e) Use of liquid helium .

167) Effect of long TE in spin echo sequence

a) Produce T2 weighted image.

b)Relatively worse SNR.

c) Does not influence acquisition time.

d) More dephasing of $M_{xy.}$

e) May limit the number of multislice acquisitions.

168) True regarding tissue contrast in Fast SE as compared to standard SE

a)Fat appears brighter than conventional SE due to increase in j-coupling effect.

b)White matter appear relatively darker due to magnetization transfer effect.

c) Signal intensity of CSF remains unaffected.

d) Accentuated susceptibility effect leading to better detection of hemorrhage.

e) More sensitive to eddy current-induced imperfections in the magnetic field gradients.

169)True regarding SNR

a)SNR is roughly proportional to magnetic field strength.

b)SNR is inversely proportional to the square root of the sampling bandwidth.

c)SNR increases according to the square of the FOV.

d) SNR increases as number of excitations increases.

e)As spatial resolution is improved, the SNR decreases in direct proportion to the volume of the voxel.

170)True regarding superconducting wire used in MRI

a) Embedded in Tin matrix.

b)The copper is the primary current conduction pathway below the critical temperature of the superconducting wire.

c) The titanium reduces a magnet s propensity to quench.

d)The critical temperature of niobium-titanium is 9k and the critical field at 4.2k is approximately 11T.

e)MRI based on conduction cooling technique requires no helium.

171) True regarding turbo STIR

a)The bright fat signal is nulled on turbo STIR.

b)T2 filtering effect of TSE less problematic.

c)Less contrast than its TSE.

d)More blurring than TSE.

e)Used in musculoskeletal imaging

172)True regarding magnetization transfer

a)T2 of the free water pool is shorter than that of the bound water pool.

b)The width in frequency of the resonance of the free pool is larger than that of the bound pool.

c)A fraction of bound pool exchanges with the free pool.

d)RF pulses are tailored to selectively saturate the resonance of the bound pool

e) Improves the resolution of small vessels in TOF angiography.

173)True regarding 2D TOF

a)Sensitive to slow blood flow.

b)incompatible with breath holding.

c) Preferred for abdominal venous studies.

d) Require thinner slice, so stronger slice select gradient than 3D TOF.

e) Better spatial resolution than 3D TOF.

174)Regarding MR signal, true statements are

a)Peak signal is proportional to proton or spine density of the voxel and also to static magnetic field.

b)Peak signal is proportional to the gyromagnetic ratio of nucleus.

c)Only mobile protons give MR signal.

d)Air in the sinuses, having no hydrogen, produces no signal and always appear black in the image.

e)Grey matter has somewhat high PD than white matter.

175) Following has very long T2

a)Compact bone and tendon .

b)Teeth and calculi.

c)Metallic clip.

d)Water

e)Fat.

176) True about short-T1 inversion recovery sequence.

a)Used for fat suppression.

b)Anti parallel spins recover more quickly in water than fat.

c) At TI (time to inversion) ,about 125ms ,Mz of fat zero.

d)At TI (about 125ms), water has some Mz.

e)T1 of water is shorter than fat .

177) True about Gd-DTPA are

a) Water- insoluble.

b) Shorten both T1 and T2 , but effect is more on T2.

c) Area of uptake is made brighter on T1 weighted image.

d) T2 weighting is used after gadolinium injection.

e) Seven unpaired electron.

178) True regarding hyperpolarized xenon(^{129}Xe)

a) Xenon does not dissolves in blood.

b) It shows large chemical shift.

c) Can be used at low fields.

d)It has good potential for MRI of the lungs and for low field angiography.

e) Potential for use in spectroscopic study.

179)True regarding Helium

a) Expensive.

b)Liquid form used.

c) Contained within fragile cryostat.

d)Replenished periodically.

e) No effect of entry of air into the system.

180) True regarding about Specific absorption ratio(SAR) are

a) SAR is the RF energy deposited per mass of tissue expressed as

Watts/gram.

b) Cornea and testes may be at risk of microwave heating.

c)Skin and rectal temperature should not exceed 0.5 degree Celsius.

d)SAR is greater for small parts than large parts.

e) SAR is greater for high static fields than low.

181) True statements about MDM are

a) Electron has a MDM of one Bohr Magneton associated with the spin.

b) Electron has MDM associated with orbital motion, depending upon shell number(K,L,M).

c) The nuclear Magneton is used to express the MDM of nuclei.

d) Gauss/Tesla is unit of magnetic field strength/ magnetic induction.

e)Nuclei with no MDM will not be detectable.

182) True regarding superconducting magnet

e) Weekly filling of liquid.

b) Quenching refers to rise of temperature of solenoid ,that is above for super conduction.

c) Copper matrix keeps the superconducting filament from melting during a quench.

d) A disturbance in the fringing fields may induce quench.

e) A large exhaust system must be in place to remove the liquid gas quickly.

183)True regarding surface coils are

a) Used as receiver and transmitter .

b) Gives better SNR.

c) Poor spatial resolution.

d) Limited field.

e) Harder to use.

184)Methods to reduce RF deposition are

a) Use of less than 180 degree refocusing pulse.

b) Parallel imaging.

c) Hyper echoes.

d) GRASE.

e)Magnetization transfer.

185)True regarding sampling bandwidth

a) Inverse relation between SNR and sampling bandwidth.

b)Low bandwidth is particularly useful in low field system.

c)With low bandwidth, larger FOV is used.

d) low bandwidth Lead to more motion and susceptibility artifact.

e) low bandwidth produce less chemical –shift artifact.

186)True statements are

a)Shielding help in containing fringe field.

c)Passive magnetic shield is done by use of large amount

of iron around the magnet or in the room wall.

c)In active shielding, a secondary coil carry current in the same direction as the main coil.

d) The field stability in superconducting MRI is governed by power supply .

e)External field fluctuation is eliminated by special superconducting moving metal coil.

187)True regarding SSFP

a) belong to both spin-echo and gradient-echo families.

b) Gradient structure is symmetrically balanced in the slice,phase-encoding,and read directions.

c) RF spoiling done.

e) In steady state, the SSFP signal is T2/T1 weighted.

e)High flip angle can be used.

188)True regarding 3D TOF

a)Cannot detect vessels with slowly moving blood such as veins and peripheral arteries.

b)Longer scan time than 2D TOF.

c)Less susceptible to turbulent signal loss(such as a stenotic segment).

e)Can grade percent stenosis within an internal carotid artery lesion.

e)Incompatible with breath holding.

189) True about permanent magnet used in MRI are

a) Made of iron and alloys of aluminium, nickel, and cobalt.

b) Heavy, about 80 tones.

c) Cheap to run.

d) Cheap to buy.

e) High power needed.

190)Regarding free induction decay, which of following are true

a)The MR signal is greatest immediately before switching off of 90degee pulse.

b)During relaxation, Mxy increases and Mz decreases .

c)During relaxation, sum vector M

spirals(beehive fashion) from transverse plane to longitudinal –z direction.

d)Spin lattice and spin-spin relaxation occurs concurrently but independently.

e)As Mz increases, strength of MR signal increases.

191) True statements about tissue characteristics are

a)T2 is always shorter than T1.

b)T2 value increases with magnetic field strength.

c)T1 value remains unaffected with magnetic field strength.

d)There are specific values for T1 and T2 for specific tissues.

e)Abnormal tissues tend to have a higher PD,T1,T2. Than normal.

192)Ways of reducing scan time are

a) Reduce TR.

b)RF pulse of shorter duration.

c) Use of larger tip angle .

d)Reducing the phase matrix.

e)Increasing the number of excitations.

193) True about Gd-DTPA

a) DTPA stands for diethylenetriaminepenta-acetic acid.

b)Shortening of T1 and T2 of adjacent hydrogen nuclei due to magnetic susceptibility effect.

c)Negative contrast agent.

d)T1 AND T2 shortening has opposite effect,so conc. used must not be great.

e)Cross blood- brain barrier.

194)Spatial resolution is increased by

a)Increase in pixel size and FOV.
b)Larger matrix.
c)Three- dimensional acquition.
d)Use of local coil.
e)Thicker slice.

195) True regarding effect of very low level of coolant in superconducting MRI

a)quenching occurs.
b) Temperature rises.
c)Loss of superconductivity.
d)Release of the stored energy.
e)Liquid helium boils off rapidly.

196) SAR is greater

a) For larger body parts.
b) For lower static magnetic field.
c) For180 degree pulse than 90 degree.
d) For SE than for GRE.
e) For high conductivity tissues (brain, live ,CSF) than low conductivity tissues(fat, bone marrow).

197) Correct data

a) One Bohr Magneton=9.27 x10^{-24}j/tesla.
b) One Tesla=10^6 Gauss.
c) Nuclear Magneton=5.05 x10^{-27}j/T.
d)MDM for proton=2.7928 x5.05 x10^{-27}j/T.
e)MDM for neutron= -1.0128 x5.05 x10^{-27} j/T.

198) True regarding electronics of MRI

a) Pulse generator can vary RF frequency to obtain the larmor frequency.

b) Pulse generator fix the pulse width.
c) Pulse generator develop the pulse sequence.
d) pulse generator and amplifier is together called Transmitter .
e) Electronics controls the gradient coils.

199) Correct acronyms are

a) FLASH – few low angle shot.
b) FEE- fast field echoes.
c)GRASS- Gradient recalled acquisition in the steady state.
d) FAST- fast acquired steady state technique.
e)FISP-fast imaging with steady precession.

200)Artefact noted in the phase encoding directions are

a) Aliasing.
b)Motion artifact.
c)Chemical artifact .
d)Truncation artifact.
e)Zipper artifact.

201) True regarding inversion recovery sequence

a)180 degree refocusing pulse is used.
b)T1 contrast is primarily dependent upon inversion time.
c) Distinguishing features of STIR is short inversion time(150 to 250ms).
d)After waiting period, MR signal is generated by fast SE pulse.
e)180 degree pulse invert magnetization fro –z axis to +z axis.

202)True regarding cross talk

a)Cross talk refers to slice

contamination by RF from the edges of adjacent slices.
b) Tissue contrast is degraded.
c)T2 weighted images are less degraded by crosstalk than T1weighted images.
d)Reduced by shorter RF.
e) Reduced by 3D.

203)True regarding SSFP

a) Saturation effect.
b) Motion sensitive.
c) Used in cardiac imaging, flow imaging.
d)Higher SNR and higher imaging efficiency compared to spoiled GRE.
e) Signal sensitivity to off-resonance is limitation of SSFP.

204)True regarding spin-lock imaging

a)provides the contrast of low fields while maintaining the large magnetic polarization and SNR of high fields.
b)Water molecules in homogenous protein solutions have spin-lattice rates that are 50% higher than that of free water at 0.5T but are five times higher at 200 micro.
c)Useful in situations where the presence of macromolecular proteins is important.
d)Typical B_{1L} is 10 micro.
e) Useful in imaging of cartilage.

205)True regarding Dark blood imaging

a)Use of double inversion technique.
b) Blood appear dark.
c)Calcified plaque has low signal .
d) Slow or recirculating flow difficult to make dark.
e) Surrounding tissue appear bright.

206)Regarding spin-lattice relaxation(longitudinal),which of following are true

a)Mz recovers .
b)T1 refers to time for Mz to recover to 63% of its maximum.
c)95% completion of recovery of Mz occurs in 3T1.
d)T1value in order of hundreds of milliseconds.
e)T1 of tissue shortens in the stronger magnetic field.

207) True regarding perfusion imaging

a) Gd remain in blood vessel during first pass.
b) Gd does not cause susceptibility effect in perfused tissues.
c) Generally T1 weighting is used after Gd injection.
d) The tracer concentration is roughly inversely proportional to the relaxation rate in normally perfused tissues.
e) Analysis of signal gain gives information on blood volume and a measurement of perfusion.

208)True regarding scan time

a)Reducing TR reduces scan time.
b)Reducing number of encodings increase scan time.
c) Reducing number of excitations reduce scan time.
d) Short scan time increase artefacts.
e) Short scan time may improve image quality.

209)True regarding magnetic field used in MRI are

a) Must be stable.
b) Must remain unaffected by ambient temperature.
C) Uniformity to 1ppm over a large volume for imaging.
d) Uniformity to 5ppm for spectroscopy.
e) Magnetic field Is usually aligned vertically in solenoid.

210) Hazards of MRI include

a) Projectile effect.
b) Displacement of aneurysm clip.
c) Burn to the patients.
d) Microwave heating.
e) Peripheral nerve stimulation.

211) True regarding MDM of nuclei are

a) The MDM of nuclei are not measured, they are calculated for each nucleus.
b) MDM of the proton or neutron is found to be different from the nuclear magneton.
c) MDM of the nuclei can be calculated by adding up the MDM of all protons and neutrons in the nucleus.
d) For spinning particles, the MDM is always along the spin axis.
e) If nucleus has no spin, it has no angular momentum and no MDM.

212) True statement is

a) Mz precess.
b) Mz can be detected.
c) FID is a very weak signal compared to the 90 degree RF pulse.
d) FID decays very fast.
e) Gradient coils and RF pulses are used to divide the patient into slices.

213) True regarding fast imaging techniques

a) A reduced flip angle allows a reasonably large Mxy while retaining a large Mz.
b) Residual Mz is proportional to the sin of the flip angle.
c) 180 degree pulse is used.
d) During negative readout gradient, there is rephasing of spins.
e) A negative readout gradient is followed by a positive readout gradient.

214) True regarding STIR

a) Distinguishing feature is use of a short TI(150 to 250ms).
b) Improved lesion conspicuity through the additive effect of T1 and T2 contrast.
c) Produce fat suppression dependent on Bo homogeneity.
d) Tissue with shorter T1 (gray matter ,csf) appear brighter than tissues with longer T1 (white matter, fat).
e) Magnitude – sensitive reconstructions of image is done.

215) True regarding FOV

a) The minimal FOV is primarily determined by the peak gradient amplitude and gradient duration.
b) Reduction in FOV decreases SNR.
c) Spatial resolution improves as the FOV is decreased.
d) Small FOV may produce wraparound artifact.
e) Low bandwidth typically permit smaller FOV.

216) Cryogenic design used in MRI

a) Vacuum vessel.

b)Thermal shields and multi layer insulation

c)Helium vessel.

d) Magnet cartridge.

e) Cryo cooler.

217)True regarding shimming

a)Process of shimming takes a few days to complete.

b)Shimming is the act of bringing the magnets homogeneity into specification.

c)Supercon shimming refers to use of superconducting correction coils.

d) Passive shimming is done by using small pieces of ferromagnetic materials.

e)High order shimming is done by use of resistive coils.

218)True regarding fast spin-echo

a)Scan time=TR x Number of phase encoded lines x number of excitations.

b) Decreases RF deposition.

c) Produce magnetization transfer effect

d)Decreased signal intensity of fat.f

e)Blurring artifact, particularly at short TE.

219)True regarding diffusion weighted imaging

a) Provides quantitative measures of the molecular motion of water in three dimensional space.

b)Used to detect acute cerebral ischemia.

c)DTI allows one to investigate the orientation of major white matter fiber tracts.

d) Signal loss depend on ADC and diffusion –sensitizing factor or b-value.

e) Diffusion weighting may be based on spin echo ,stimulated echo, SSFP.

220)True regarding phase – contrast imaging

a)Moving spins develop a phase shift with respect to stationary spins as they move in a pair of opposing magnetic field gradients.

b)Flow- encoding gradient is intentionally applied along any axis.

c) Only motion in the flow encoding direction results in a net phase shift.

d)PC utilizes the magnitude information to obtain MR angiogram, images of directional flow, and flow quantification.

e) May evaluate the physiological significance of a diseased vessel.

221)Regarding T1, which of following are true

a)Mxy recovers.

b)T1 is time for Mz to recover to 63%of its maximum value.

c)After three time constants (3T1) ,recovery is 87% complete.

d)T1 value is of order of many hundreds of milliseconds.

e)T1 of tissue lengthens in stronger magnetic field.

222.True regarding MR contrast

a. gadolinium chelates lowers localized T1, T2 and T2*

b. Gd-chelates do not cross the intact blood–brain barrier

c. SPIOs is primarily used for liver pathology

d. blueberry juice may act as negative MR contrast agent

e. blueberry juice may be used in MR cholangiopancreatography

223) The static magnetic field is not perfectly uniform because of

a)Magnetic field gradient.

b)Imperfections in the magnet.

c)The introduction of patient.

d)Earth s magnetic field.

e)Gravitational pull .

224)True regarding tip angle

a)15 degree pulse produces 25%of usual Mxy but leaves 97%of Mz.

b)The stronger the initial RF pulse and the longer its duration, the greater tip angle.

c)The greater the tip angle, the greater the T2 weighting.

d)For T2 and PD weighting, use >70 degree tip angle.

e)The shorter TR is, compared withT1,the smaller is the optimum tip angle.

225.True regarding high tesla MR

a.increased magnetic susceptibility contrast (useful for depicting nuclei within the brainstem or fMRI responses)

b.greater resolution between resonance peaks in spectroscopy (potentially helpful for water/fat imaging) and

c.decrease in tissue T1s (prolonged blood signal and better background suppression for time-of-flight angiography).

d. increased metallic foreign-body

artefact

e dereased chemical shift artifact

226) True regarding gradient (recalled) echo(GRE) are

a) Use of short TR (typically 15ms).

b)Use of reduced strength and tip angle(<90 degree) as compared with SE echo.

c)Use of positive and negative frequency encoding gradient.

d)GRE does not eliminate effect inhomogeneities in the static field, so image is T2* weighted.

e)GRE does not compensate for magnetic susceptibility.

227) True about arterial spin labeling

a) Use of spin inversion technique by applying off resonance RF.

b)In spin- labeled image ,blood-water magnetization is in same state from that of tissue-water magnetization.

c)In controlled image ,blood- water magnetization – is in different state from that of tissue-water magnetization.

d) No inversion is applied in control image.

e) subtractting the two images give the perfusion image.

228)True regarding aliasing in MRI

a)Aliasing is a sign that FOV is too small.

b) Wrap-round of image in frequency- encoding direction.

c) Design of electronic circuit to

suppress aliasing in phase encoding direction.
d) Increase FOV to reduce aliasing.
e) Use of coil matching to FOV.

229) True regarding fringe field in MRI

a) Fringe field refers to the magnetic field lines spread widely outside the solenoid.
b) Stronger is the magnetic field, smaller is the fringe field.
c) The fringe field of a permanent magnet is very large .
d) The fringe field is reduced by an iron shroud.
e) Shimming coil do not reduce fringe field.

230) contraindications of MRI are

a) Aneurysm clip.
b) Ferrous foreign bodies especially eye.
c) Joint prostheses.
d) Dental prostheses.
e) Cardiac pacemaker.

231) Following isotope has nuclear spin ½

a) ^{1}H.
b) ^{13}C.
c) ^{19}F.
d) ^{2}H.
e) ^{14}N .

232) True regarding slice selection gradient

a) Typical gradient coil magnetic field strength are .2 to 1 gauss/cm (0.00002 to 0.0001 T/cm).
b) The frequency of the RF pulse selects slice thickness.

c) The bandwidth of the RF pulse selects the location of slice thickness.
d) Coils are resistive electromagnet.
e) Clicking sound heard during MRI is produced by the switching of gradient coils.

233) True regarding history of MRI

a) MR imaging was first demonstrated on two small tubes of water by Paul lauterbur in 1972.
b) Fourier transform is the basis of most imaging modalities.
c) 1946 is year in which MR was discovered.
d) MR phenomenon was independently discovered by Felix Bloch and Edward Purcell.
e) Felix and Purcell shared the Nobel Prize for physics in 1946.

234) True regarding STIR

a) Inversion time to suppress fat is of the order of 150ms.
b) Increases the conspicuity of lesions embedded in fat(lymph node, orbit).
c) Can distinguish fat from blood products.
d) STIR augment signal in contrast enhanced setting.
e) Suppress fat independent of Bo homogeneity.

235) True regarding matrix

a) For a given FOV, a 256 x256 matrix has twice the spatial resolution than that of a 128 x128 matrix.
b) The imaging time is proportional to the number of phase –encoding

steps.

c)Changing the matrix size along the frequency-encoding direction changes scan time.

d)Decrease in matrix size minimize truncation artifact.

e)In rectangular field of view, spatial resolution can be improved despite decrease in matrix size.

236..True regarding historical perspective of MRI

a. spin-warp imaging by Edelstein

b. Functional MRI (fMRI) of the brain was introduced by Ogawa et al in 1992, and developed by Rosen et

c.SMASH introduced by Sodickson et al in 1997

d. SENSE introduced by Pruessmann et al in 1999

e. Bloch and Purcell were jointly awarded the Nobel Prize for Physics in 1952

337) True regarding gradient coil

a) Gradient amplitude defines the minimum field strength of a gradient system(millitesla/meter).

b)Gradient slew rate is the rate of change of the gradient strength.(T/m/s).

c) Gradient duty cycle describes the percentage of time the gradient subsystem can provide minimum gradient strength pulse sequence waveforms.

d)X and Y gradient coils(cylindrical) has different geometry than the Z gradient(saddle-shaped).

e)Maxwell coil is used as Z gradient coil while Golay coils is used as X and Y gradient coils.

238)True regarding incoherent GRE

a)The spoiler gradient is applied at the end of the readout.

b)The spoiler gradient disperses any residual longitudinal magnetization that remains after the signal has been read.

c)The flip angle that produces the minimum signal for the given TR and T1 is known as the Ernst angle.

d)A flip angle larger than the Ernst angle produces better T1 contrast.

e) For proton density- weighted images, a smaller flip angle is desirable.

239)True regarding contrast

a)The contrast typically makes diseased tissue appear brighter (or in some cases darker) than the surrounding tissue.

b)The first approved contrast agent,Gd DTPA appeared in 1988.

c)The effect of MRI contrast agent is observed directly .

d)MRI contrast agent perturbs in some way the magnetic properties of hydrogen.

e) The diagnostic potential of paramagnetic agents was first demonstrated in patients by Young, using Gd DTPA.

240) True regarding PC angiography

a)Phase shift is inversely proportional to velocity of blood flow.

b) Phase shift is proportional to the gradient strength.

c) Phase shift is proportional to the gradient strength.

d) Choose a velocity encoding range

(V_{ENC}) that is slightly lower than the maximal anticipated velocity in the vessel of interest.

e) Velocity aliasing shows gradual transition of phase in the vessel.

241.True regarding historical perspective of MRI

a. The phenomenon of 'nuclear induction'(nuclear magnetic resonance (NMR) was described independently by Bloch and Purcell and their colleagues in 1946

b.Bloch and Purcell were jointly awarded the Nobel Prize for Physics in 1952

c. Damadian noted that in vitro elevated MR relaxation times in animal tumours (1971)

d. . Human in vivo images were first published in 1977 by Mansfield and Maudsley Damadian et al, and Hinshaw et al

e. Multiplanar imaging ability was first demonstrated by Hawkes et al in 1980

242)True statements about typical relaxation times(ms)T1 and T2 of tissues in a field of 1T are

a)Fat   250/ 80
b)White matter   650 /90.
c)Grey matter   800/100.
d)Liver   400/40.
e)Water   3000/150 .

243) True statement regarding spin echo sequence are

a)180 degree pulse is called refocusing pulse.

b)Each 90 degree pulse is followed by 180 pulse.

c)180 degree pulse is used to remove systemic magnetic field inhomogeneities.

d)Rephasing of Mxy starts immediately after 90 degree pulse.

e)Dephasing of Mxy starts just after 180 degree pulse.

244)True regarding GRE are

a)No use of 180 degree pulse.

b) The positive gradient pulse rephrases the spins while negative one dephases spins.

c)The positive gradient pulse(x) duration equals the negative gradient pulse(x^1).

d)The peak of MR signal appears at the middle of x-gradient pulse.

e)Moving blood appears dark.

245) True regarding Magnetization transfer

a) Substantial additional RF power deposition.

b) Useful in intracranial angiography.

c) Improves conspicuity of brain metastases.

d)Increased MT rate in multiple sclerosis.

e)Use of off-resonance RF pulse.

246)True regarding diffusion imaging(DWI)

a) Use of EPI or fast GRE sequences.

b)Application of two large gradient pulses after each RF excitation .

C)Sensitivity weighting factor depend on only time of the diffusion gradient.

d)High signal appears from tissues with restricted movement DWI.

e) Signal attenuation is directly

related to the apparent(or effective) diffusion coefficient divided by sensitivity weighting factor.

247)True regarding motion artefacts in MRI

a)Cause blurring or smearing of the image.
b) Produce only one ghost image.
c) Effects usually apparent in the frequency encoding direction.
d) May produce multiple ghost images of abdominal aorta .
e) Heart motion , breathing, pulasatile flow in arteries may produce ghost image.

248)True regarding fringe field

a) Affect some watches.
b) Destroy data on CD.
C) Distort nearby video displays.
d)Affect photomultipliers.
e) Effect minimized by use of iron shielding.

249) Effects that are against use of higher magnetic field.

a) Increase in T1, necessitating a longer TR and imaging time.
b) Greater cost of magnet .
c) Hard to make magnetic field uniform.
d) Stronger fringe field, affecting equipment in adjacent areas.
e) Increased chemical artifact.

250) Following isotope has nuclear spin ½

a) ^{1}H.
b) ^{13}C.
c)^{23} Na.
d) ^{27}Al.
e)^{31} P.

251)True regarding slice width and crosstalk

a) Pulse width of 4258 kHz will select 1cm wide slice(1T field and gradient of 1Gauss/cm).
b) Slice crosstalk refers to signal from outside of the intended slice volume.
c) Slice crosstalk is due to fact that RF pulse is precise in frequency.
d) Gap in slices is intended to overcome slice crosstalk.
e) Slice crosstalk enhance the image quality.

252) True regarding history of MRI

a)Lauterbur shared the Nobel Prize for medicine with Peter Mansfield in 2003.
b) Peter Mansfield devised echo-planar imaging(1977) and used it to demonstrate the first MR clinical image.
c)Abrikosov ,V.Ginzburg and A Legget shared the Nobel prize in physics in 2003 for theory of superconductivity.
d) J Henning designated the improved spin-echo sequence as RARE.
e)Ernst introduced Fourier transform to MR.

253)True regarding FLAIR

a)Fluids tend to have the longest T1 values of the tissue components.
b)T1of CSF is of several seconds.
c) Fluid signal can be suppressed by using long inversion time 750to 2000ms.
d)T1 FLAIR can produce better

contrast between gray and white matter and better suppression than T1 SEsequence.

e)T2 FLAIR makes periventricular lesions bright and suppress csf signal.

254)Effect of imaging at 3T

a)Improved SNR and spatial resolution

b)less robust fat suppression.

c) Less chemical shift.

d) Less power deposition.

e)Reduced dose of paramagnetic contrast.

255)True regarding transmit chain

a)The coil used to produce linear fields (B₁) is known as quadrature transmit coils.

b)Linear polarized B_1 fields require twice the amount of RF power than circular polarized B_1 fields to flip the spin to a given angle.

c) Circular polarization is twice as efficient as linear polarization.

d) Birdcage RF coil generates a B_1 field on the transverse plane.

e)3Db hybrid splitter is a transmit chain component.

256)True regarding steady-state free precession GRE

a)Recycling of longitudinal magnetization that persist after readout.

b)There is an extra phase-encoding gradient ,of opposite sign to the regular phase-encoding gradient.

c)The difference in contrast behavior between spoiled and SSFP

GRE is manifested only conditions of TR>>T2 and large flip angle.

d) Fluid appear bright.

E) Moving fluid does not appear uniformly bright.

257)True statement

a)Diamagnetic substance has net electron spin.

b) Paramagnetic has no net electron spin.

c) Paramagnetic substance has even number of electron.

d) Contrast agents possess net electron spin.

e)Gd has five unpaired electron.

258) True regarding display in PC angiography

a)Net phase shift(velocity map) is used for velocity and flow volume calculations.

b) Complex difference image (the magnitude of vector difference) is used mainly for scout imaging.

c) Speed image is not ideal for anatomic depiction of vascular anatomy.

d)There is information regarding flow direction in speed image .

e) Flow encoding is performed in only one direction in velocity map.

259)True statements about typical relaxation time T1 of tissues in a field of 1T are

a)Fat 650.

b)Kidney 550.

c)Csf 2000.

d)Bone and teeth very short.

e)Grey matter 800

260)Difference of GRE as compared to spin echo

a)No use of 180 degree pulse.

b)Does not eliminate effect of magnetic field inhomogeneities of static field.

c)Use of reduced strength and tip angle of RF pulse.

d)Use of gradient pulse to rephrase .

e) Gives T2* image.

261)True about echo planar imaging are

a)Extremely rapid form of GRE.

b) Produce 50ms snapshot.

c)Use of standard (90,180) SE sequence.

d) Frequency encoding gradient is continually reversed as fast as possible.

e) Phase encoding gradient is switched on and off just before each echo.

262)True about magnetic susceptibility effect of GRE

a) GRE more sensitive than SE to magnetic field inhomogeneities.

b) May produce artifact at ferromagnetic implants, at air-soft tissue, bone- soft- tissue interface

c) 2D GRE is more sensitive than 3D GRE

d) May produce signal loss, geometric distortion and zebra artifact.

e) Useless in detection of hemorrhagic lesion.

263)True about diffusion gradient in DWI

a) Gradient pulse are applied before RF excitation.

b) Gradients used must be weak.

c) The gradient pulses effectively

cancel if spins do not move while moving spins undergo phase shift.

d)Tissues with normal random thermal motion/diffusion enhances the signal.

e) DWI may give quantitative assessment of tissue integrity and connectivity.

264)True about ghost images are

a)Usually apparent in phase encoding direction.

b)Cardiac motion may produce multiple ghost images.

c) The faster the motion, less spacing of the ghost images.

d)Cardiac trigger can reduce cardiac motion artifact.

e)Gradient moment rephrasing is a way to suppress motion artefacts.

265) Factors against use of high magnetic field

a) Longer imaging time.

b) Worsening of motion and susceptibility artifact.

c) More RF heating.

d) More potential of hazard to patient.

e) More cost.

266)True regarding patient screening for MRI

a) History of implants ,especially pacemaker.

b)Surgical history.

c) Functional disorder.

d) Allergy of contrast agent.

e) Weight of patient.

267) True statement regarding nucleus

a) The nucleus can come in exact

alignment with the magnetic field.

b) The up orientation has slightly higher energy than that of down orientation.

c) All nuclei of tissue participate in the NMR signal.

d) The ratio of up/down orientation is determined by energy difference between states, the magnetic field and the temperature.

e) Torque (magnetic field) remaining after orientation of nuclei is responsible for the MDM·sprecessing about the magnetic field.

268) True statements are

a) Phase encoding is the first step in dividing a slice into voxels.

b) At the end of phase encoding, all Mxy are in the same phase.

c) Frequency gradient is the readout gradient.

d) The way the RF coil and gradients fields are turned on and off is called a pulse sequence.

e) Coils are resistive electromagnet.

269)True regarding protons and neutrons

a) They intrinsically possess angular momentum.

b)The intrinsic angular momentum of a neutron or proton is called spin.

c)They possess magnetic dipole moment that is inversely proportional to their intrinsic spin.

d) Gyromagnetic ratio=magnetic moment/spin

e) Spin of ^{23}Na is ½.

270)True regarding Gradient-

echo

a)No use of 180 degree refocusing pulse.

b)Flip angle usually less than 90 degree.

c) Use of much shorter TR (of the order of 3 to 250ms)

d) Scan time dramatically reduced

e)Tissue contrast relate to flip angle and spoiling.

271) True regarding phase contrast imaging

a)Water protons precess 3.5ppm more rapidly than fat protons.

b)Water and fat signal oscillate in and out of phase with a periodicity of 3.4ms/T

c)Fat and water is in phase when TE is in odd multiple of 3.4ms.

d) Fat water signal modulation occurs in SE sequence.

e)Opposed images are readily identified by dark borders surrounding organs at fat water interface

272) True regarding MRS imaging are

a) Gyromagnetic ratio of zero can produce MR signal. f

b)^{16}0,^{14}N,^{12}C possess nuclear magnetism.

c)^{31}P has higher gyromagnetic ratio(17.2MHz) than that of ^{1}H.

d) Magnetic field should be uniform to better than 10ppm.

e) Only phase encoding gradient can be used.

273)True regarding balanced coherent gradient echo

a) Symmetrical gradient structure

that eliminates phase shift caused by motion.

b)Bile, blood and csf,fat appear dark .

c) Ideal for scout imaging.

d)Using cardiac gating, it is method of choice for cine MRI.

e)Tendency to have bright stripes in the image.

274)Correct matching of paramagnetic metal and unpaired electron

a)Iron(ii) 5

b)Preseodymium 2

c)Gadolinium(iii) 7.

d)Dysprosium(iii) 5.

e)Holmium (iii) 4.

275)True regarding phase contrast angiography

a) Short TR (30-40ms).

b)Short TE (8ms or less).

c)Small FA (20-30 degree).

d) Vessel appear bright.

e) Small voxel.

276)True order of T1 value of different tissue

a)Fat<grey matter<csf.

b)Liver<fat<white matter.

c) Grey matter<water<csf.

d)Bone and teeth<grey matter<csf.

e)White matter<grey matter<csf.

277) True statements regarding slice in MRI

a)The slice thickness is reduced by increasing the gradient of magnetic field.

b)The slice thickness is reduced by increasing the RF bandwidth.

c)Thinner slice produce more partial volume effect.

d)Cross talk can be prevented by leaving a gap between slices.

e)The slice orientation depends upon the physical gradient axis(z-axis gives a transverse slice).

278)True about echo planar imaging

a) PD,T2 weighted image is obtained by using short or long effective TE.

b) TI weighting is not possible.

c) whole brain can be imaged in about 2-3s.

d) used for functional imaging, real-time cardiac imaging, perfusion or diffusion imaging.

e) Artefact is not a problem.

279)True about functional MRI

a) Oxyhaemoglobin is paramagnetic.

b) Deoxyhaemoglobin is diamagnetic.

c) Deoxyhaemoglobin produces magnetic field inhomogeneities, increasing T2*

d) At rest tissues have roughly equal amount of oxy and deoxyhaemoglobin.

e)During activity, oxyhaemoglobin increase.

280) Factors in favor of high magnetic field are

a) larger signal.

b) larger SNR.

C) Special applications.

d)Less hazard to patient.

e)Less chemical artifact.

281) Relevant steps for MRI

a) Removal of hairpin.

b) Removal of jewellery.

c) Remove eye make-up for brain mri.

d) Take weight for SAR.

e) Allergy history.

282) True about Larmor frequency are

a) The frequency of precession is known as the Larmor frequency.

b) Larmor frequency= gyromagnetic field x magnetic field /2pi.

c) Gyromagnetic ratio is the ratio of MDM to the nuclear spin angular momentum.

d) Gyromagnetic ratio is a unique value for each type of nucleus.

e) Planck's constant=6.6×10^{-34}j.sec.

283) True about spin echo sequence

a)Slice selection gradient is applied slightly before 90 degree pulse.

b)Slice select gradient is not removed during at the end of 90 degree pulse.

c) Frequency encoding gradient is turned on during echo detection.

d) FID is not detected.

e)The time of echo is determined by the time between the 90 degree and 180 degree.

284)True statements are

a)The motion of the spin about the axis of an externally applied magnetic field is called precession.

b) Frequency of precession= gyromagnetic ratio / applied field strength.

c)When spin system is in thermal equilibrium, slightly more spins are in the higher energy state.

d) Thermal equilibrium magnetization (Mo) is directly proportional to static magnetic field (Bo).

e) Thermal equilibrium magnetization (Mo) is inversely proportional to temperature.

285) True regarding GRE

a)With incoherent GRE,transverse magnetization after signal readout is refocused.

b)Incoherent GRE primarily yield T1W and proton density weighted image.

c)FLASH,SPGR,TIFFE are coherent GRE sequences.

d)Transverse magnetization is dispersed after readout in incoherent GRE.

e)Tissue contrast is a function of T1/T2 Incoherent GRE.

286)True about Magnetization transfer contrast

a) Invisible spin associated with large proteins ,membranes.

b) Invisible spins has very short T2(<0.1ms) and cannot be seen at any typically used TE.

c) Off resonance MT RF pulses saturates the mobile proton.

d) Restricted proton becomes saturated due to exchange of magnetization between two pools.

e) In MT contrast , the signal from mobile protons increase.

287) True about multislice imaging

a) Take advantage of the long

waiting time required by the TR interval.

b) Both TR and TE determine number of slices.

c) A new slice can be excited before detection of echo from the previous slice.

d) Total scan time is tremendously shortened.

e) Gap is used to eliminate the overlap area.

288)True about MRI are

a)Z-axis along the length of the patient.

b)Magnetic field strength usually between 0.15 to 3T.

c)1T is about 10000 times greater than the earth's magnetic field.

d)Static magnetic field B highly uniform.

e)Patient become highly magnetized inside the coil.

289)True regarding EPI

a)Proposed by Mansfield and Pykett.

b)Fastest clinically useful technique.

c)Image acquisition time of the order of one tenth of a second.

d)Useful in perfusion ,diffusion and f MRI.

e) Ghost images due to breathing and cardiac pulsation seen.

290)True regarding different forms of magnetism

a)Diamagnetic always align parallel to external field.

b)Paramagnetic align ant parallel to external magnetic field.

c)Ferromagnetic material does not possess magnetism outside the magnetic field.

d)Relative magnetic susceptibility of supraparamagnetic is +5000.

e)Examples of paramagnetic materials are Gd, and molecular oxygen.

291)True regarding PCA

a) Image intensity is related to magnitude

b) Reflection of blood inflow in the slice.

c) Near complete background elimination.

d) better detection of small vessel.

e)All stationary materials , fat , metheglobin are eliminated.

292)True about T1W are

a)TR and TE are both long.

b)TR used is about the same as the average T1 of tissue of interest (300-800).

c) TE (approx.15ms) is used to reduce effect of T2.

d)Shorter is T1, stronger is signal and brighter the pixel.

e)Fat is bright while water and csf are dark.

293)True statements regarding K-SPACE are

a)A spatial frequency domain in the computer

b)Store data from every signal in a selected slice

c) Has axes corresponding to frequency and phase.

d)The number of lines filled in the k space exceeds number of encodings in the sequence.

e)Completely filled k space can be processed into image.

294) True about echo planar imaging

a) Resolution ,echo strength, and signal to noise ratio is not compromised.
b) No need of strong magnetic field.
c) Need of very high gradients and very fast switching.
d)Induction of small, unwanted currents in nearby metallic structures.
e) Active shielding of the gradient coil reduce artefacts.

295)True about f MRI are

a) Acquire images of the brain during activity and compare with at-rest images.
b)Blood oxygen level is the basis
c)Use of EPI.
d) Deoxyhaemoglobin increases T2*.
e) Oxyhaemoglobin is paramagnet attention

296) True about magnetic susceptibility

a) Noted at the interface between tissues and air in lungs ,sinuses.
b) At location of bleeding.
c) Due to inhomogeneities in local magnetic field.
d) Always lead to decrease in MR signal .
e) More evident in GRE sequences.

297)True regarding coil are

a)Shim coil and gradient coil carry AC current.

b)Shim coil make magnetic field uniform.
c) Shim coil produce loud bang
d)Steeper the slice –select gradient , the thicker the slice.
e) Steeper the frequency encoding ,smaller the FOV

298) True regarding Quenching

a)Controlled quenching needed in case of fire.
b) Accidental quenching may cause frostbite and suffocation.
c) Non-ferrous carbon dioxide extinguishers used in case of fire.
d)Start external venting system.
e) Break glass window to equalize pressure.

299) True regarding Larmor frequency

a) Each type of nucleus precess at a unique frequency in a given magnetic field.
b) A given nucleus precess at different frequency when in different magnetic field.
c) Larmor frequency of Hydrogen nucleus (proton)=42.58 MHz/T.
d)Larmor frequency of ^{31}P= 3.08 MHz/T.
e) Larmor frequency of ^{27}Al = 11.09 MHz/T.

300) True regarding spin echo sequence

a) The time interval between 90 degree and 180 degree pulse is called the TR interval.
b) The TE is the time from the middle of the 90 degree pulse to the peak of the detected echo

c)TE is much shorter (0.03s-0.15s) than TR.

d) TR interval varies between 0.5s and 2-3s.

e) Time for acquiring image in spin echo=phase encoding steps X TE x averages.

301)True statements are

a) The angle between the z-axis and M at the end of the RF pulse is called the flip angle for the pulse.

b)Nutation refers to the spiraling movement of M toward the z plane.

c) Excitation pulse refers to RF pulse used to convert transverse magnetization into longitudinal magnetization.

d)Inversion pulse (180degree) is used to move the magnetization from the positive to the negative axis.

e)Refocusing pulse (180 degree) refers to pulse used to flip the transverse magnetization about the axis along which the RF pulse is applied.

302)True regarding balanced steady state free precession,SSFP

a)Flip angle relatively large(50 to 90 degree)

b) Beneficial in ultrafast acquisitions

c) sensitive to motion artifact.

d) Fluid and fat appear dark.

e) preferred sequence for cine cardiac imaging.

303)True about MT contrast

a)Mobile protons resonate over wide range of resonance frequencies. b)Restricted protons resonate over narrow range of frequencies.

c)MT pulses primarily affect tissue that contain both mobile and invisible protons(brain,liver,muscle)

d) CSF ,urine has paucity of restricted protons and show minimal signal change.

e)MT pulses has pronounced effect on fat or that of Gd –enhanced tissue.

304)True related to inversion recovery

a)The time between inversion and excitation pulse(TI) appropriate to null a species is related to its T1 as TI=0.693T1

b)As fat suppression technique, STIR is more robust than the chemical shift method.

c)STIR has stringent requirement of static field homogeneity.

d)STIR is not susceptible to susceptibility gradient.

e)Specialized adiabatic RF pulses are generally used for inversion because they are insensitive to B_1.

305)True regarding Single-shot EPI

a) All data collected after one RF excitation.

b) Application of rapidly oscillating gradient along the readout direction.

c)Pronounced T1 Weighting.

d) Helpful in characterization of short T1, short T2 lesions such as cyst and hemangioma.

e) TR is essentially infinite.

306) True regarding contrast agents

a) All contrast agents shorten both

T1 and T2.

b) Positive contrast agent dominantly lower T2 and increase signal.

c) Negative contrast agent largely increase the 1/T2 of tissue selectively and cause a reduction in signal intensity.

d)Large iron oxide particles are example of negative contrast agent.

e)Gd based contrasts are example of positive contrast agent.

307) True regarding PCA

a) Provide MIP of larger volume

b) Suited for imaging of slow flow as vein and large aneurysm.

c) Can detect flow of CSF.

d) Used to perform flow quantification and to obtain velocity-time curve in pulsatile flow.

e) Shorter time than TOF.

308)True about T2W are

a)TR and TE are both short.

b)TE used is about the same as the average T2 of tissue of interest. (90-140)

c)TR (1000-2000) is used to reduce effect of T1 on contrast.

d)Longer is T2, stronger is signal and brighter the pixel.

e) water and csf appear darker than fat.

309) True about the central part of k space are

a)Data from shallow encoding gradient.

b)High spatial frequencies.

c) Less detail.

d)Stronger signal.

e)Both high and low frequencies.

310)True about gradient for imaging

a) For coronal plane, y-gradient is used for slice selection.

b) For sagittal plane, x-gradient is used for slice selection.

c) For axial plane , z- gradient is used for slice selection.

d)For coronal oblique plane, slice selection is applied in the x-and y-gradient simultaneously.

e) Generally speaking , the phase encoding gradient is best applied along the longer dimension of the patient anatomy.

311) Regarding MRS imaging

a) provides frequency spectrum of tissues based on molecular and chemical composition.

b) a nuclide must have low gyromagnetic ratio.

c)^{1}H is easiest to image.

d) low magnetic field(<1T) is needed.

e) only phase encoding gradient can be used.

312)True about chemical shift artifact

a) noted in phase –encoding direction .

b) fat has slightly lower resonant frequency.

c) noted around kidney , optic nerve .

d) noted at a margin of vertebral bodies.

e) higher static field produce reduces chemical shift.

313) Effect of increasing TR are

a) SNR decreases.
b) More slices possible.
c) Shortening of scan time.
d) Decrease T1 contrast.
e) Increase of both T1 AND T2 contrast.

314) True statements are

a) Spin up state has higher energy than the spin down state.
b) Transition radiation refers to the energy absorbed by the nucleus when it flips from the lower energy state to the higher energy state.
c) Radiationless transition refers to energy transfer to lattice and usually produce heat.
d) The Larmor frequency of precession is exactly twice to frequency of radiation absorbed in a transition from one spin state to another.
e) Radio frequency range from 1KHz to 100MHz.

ANSWER
Magnetic Resonance Imaging

1)acd

The excess nuclei in the lower energy state give a net MDM component along the field.Magnetization vector can precess about magnetic field if the magnetization and the magnetic field are not parallel.

2)ade

In PD weighted image ,as short as possible TE(15ms) used is to reduce the effect of T2.Long TR (1000-3000ms) is used to reduce effect of T1 on contrast.

3)bc

Upper and lower part of k space contain data from steeper encoding gradient and has low signal intensity.

4)bce

In volume imaging ,a shallow gradient is used to select thick slice, enough to include whole volume to be imaged. Data processing requirements are increased.

5)abc

Magnetic susceptibility can be reduced by use of SE sequence.Truncation can be reduced by increasing phase encoding.

6)abcde

7)ade

Decrease in slice thickness increase spatial resolution and partial volume effects lessen.

8)abce

Hydrogen is abundant in water and in fat.

9)abc

In multiecho imaging ,the signal strength of the echo decreases with lengthening of TE time. Images obtained from echoes with longer TE intervals will contain more noises but show greater image contrast.

10)abd

$T2^*$ incorporates both the tissue T2 value and the contribution from field inhomogeneities. $T2^*$ is due to reversible dephasing.

11)acd

MP-RAGE is an inversion recovery magnetization-prepared 3D GRE acquisition.

12)ace

Flow compensation increase signal intensity from flowing blood and CSF. Used in TOF MR angiography.

13)ace

At 1.5T, hydrogen nuclei in fat molecules precess at approximately 210Hz below hydrogen nuclei in water.CHESS require stringent static magnetic field.

14)bde

In EPI breathing or cardiac pulsation does not cause ghost

artifact in single shot artifact.N/2 ghosts propagate along the phase encoding direction.

15)acde

Transverse relaxivity is larger than the longitudinal relaxivity.

16)bcde

In CE MRA, contrast (Gd) is used to shorten T1 of blood.

17)abcde

18)abde

Higher slew rate (gradient magnetic field change per unit time.) in EPI reduce susceptibility and $T2^*$ filtering effects.

19)bce

Contrast agent like Gd-DTPA contain an 8-coordinate ligand binding site to Gadolinium. Octadentate ligand has role in excretion of contrast.

20)abcd

In CE MRA is insensitive to saturation.

21)bcd

Hydrogen has single proton and has large magnetic moment.

22)ade

Tissue with long T1 give small signal and dark pixel.Air and cortical bone appear black in all images.

23)abce

With steep gradient, spins are evenly distributed and the signal will be zero.

24)abc

3-D FT is used to decode the information. The three-dimensional data can be reformatted to produce images of a series of very thin contiguous slices (no gap) in any orientation with no cross talk.

25)acde

In ^{31}P MRS,MR signal is several orders of magnitude less than that of ^{1}H.

26)cd

Zipper artifact refers to a central line across the middle of the image,usually in the phase encoding direction.

27)acd

RF(transmitter/receiver) coils produce magnetic field at right angles to main magnetic field. Body coil is used to transmit RF pulse and also for receiving signal

28) a

Increase in matrix leads to smaller pixel and improved spatial resolution.Decrease in matrix increases SNR and shorten scan time.

29)bce

All MRI signals are a measure of the value of Mxy. Relative spin density is greater in grey matter than the white matter.

30)abcde

31)ade

TurboFLASH give excellent T1 contrast and Scan time is of the order of 1 second.

32) bcde

During quenching, helium gas may expand 25 to 400 times its original volume.

33) bcde

FLASH or Spoiled GRASS is used for fast T1 weighting.

34) abe

Fat suppression is essential in single shot EPI to overcome chemical shift artifact . Chemical shift artifact is many times larger than the standard sequences.

35)abcd

36)ade

Gd shorten both T1 and T2. Gd^{+3} itself is toxic.

37)abde

Re-emitted radio waves are used for reconstruction of images in MRI

38)abde

In T1W images,white matter appears brighter than grey matter.

39) bce

FOV may be increased by use of less steep field gradient . Imaging time =number of excitations x number of phase encoding steps x TR.

40)acde

SMASH and SENSE are partially parallel imaging techniques.

41)acde

^{16}O has no gyromagnetic ratio and so it is not MR active nuclide.

42) abe

Truncation artifact is more likely in the phase encoding direction ,reduced by reducing the FOV.

43)ab

Surface coil receive signal effectively from a depth equal to the coil radius. They pick up larger signal and less noise. They allow smaller voxels and give better resolution and have a smaller FOV.

44)b

Increase of FOV increases SNR and aliasing artefacts becomes less likely. Decrease of FOV improves spatial resolution.

45)abc

Tissue with a short T1 recover signal strength rapidly after a 90 degree pulse. Tissue with a long T1 recover signal strength slowly after a 90 degree pulse.

46) b

SE is also called Hahn echo. Water and most of biological tissues(diamagnetic materials) have a small negative (in the order of few ppm) magnetic susceptibility.GRE is much more sensitive than SE to magnetic susceptibility .Chemical shift for hydrogen nuclei in fat is 3.5ppm less than that for hydrogen nuclei in water.

47)abd

HASTE is not sensitive to cardiac and respiratory motion and blurring is less concern in MR urography and cholangiography.

48) abcd

Low operating cost of resistive magnet is high

49.

In TurboFLASH, the Ernst angle is small, a single inversion pulse is applied before acquiring all of the image data (k-space)

50)ad

The center of k-space consists of data acquired during the weakest phase encoding gradients. The data in the center of k-space controls image contrast. The data in the outer part of k-space controls image detail.

51)bde

FID refers to the signal that is measured just after an excitation pulse. Free in FID refers to fact that after the B_1 field is turned off at the end of the RF pulse, the magnetization processes freely in the applied static magnetic field.

52)cde

Gd contrast are all Very hydrophilic. And have similar relaxivities.

53)de

MS-325 AND B-22956 bind reversibly with albumin.

54)bd

Proton spins continuously. Solenoid coil of MRI carries DC current.Earths magnetic field is about 50micro tesla.

55)ade

Generally speaking , tissues with long T1 also has long T2. Images cannot be weighted for both T1 and T2 .

56)bde

Increasing the number of excitations reduce noise. On tissue movement ,signals will be attributed to the wrong pixels in the phase-encoding direction of k space.

57) a

The resonant frequency of the proton is about 3 ppm more in fat than in water. A water plus fat image is obtained by setting the TE they are exactly in phase. A water minus fat image is obtained by slightly delaying the TE until they are exactly out of phase.

58)ace

In phased array coils there are multiple receiver coils whose signals are received individually and produce less noise.

59) ade

Local coil increase SNR and decreases aliasing.

60)abcde

61) ade

T1 value of fat is minimally influenced by magnetic field strength. Percent decrease in Mxy depends on T2 time of the tissue and TE of the spin- echo sequence.

62)acde

At the is center ,magnetic field from the gradient coil is zero

63)abcde

64)bce

Permanent magnet produce low and mid-field(</- .05T) magnetic field and low fringe field.

65)abce

Turbo STEAM capture magnetization stored along z-axis.

66)abcd

The data in the center contain low spatial frequencies.

67) abc

Magnevist,Gadoteridol.,Gadodiamide are not a macomolecularGd chelates.

68) abd

1T is about 20000 times greater than the earth's magnetic field. Patient become slightly magnetized inside the coil.

69)bd

The steeper a gradient, greater the power consumed by the gradient coil. Increasing the matrix makes no difference to total scan time. Motion artefacts occurs in phase encoding direction.

70)abcde

71) abe

72)ae

Permanent magnet needs

temperature control, cannot be turned off in emergency and has low operating cost.

73)abe

In FISP,the phase of RF is alternated on successive excitations. The phase encoding rewinding table is used.

74)abd

Half Fourier reduce scan time nearly two fold, decrease SNR and increase sensitivity to motion.

75)abcd

Gd-DTPA is not a liver agent.

76)abde

In MRS, in order to receive same signal much larger voxel is needed in MRS.

77)ade

Slightly more magnetic dipoles orient in spin up direction than spin down orientation and mri depends on detecting this small difference in spin orientation of magnetic dipoles.

78) ade

Slice select gradient is switched on during the application of the RF application. Phase encoding gradient is applied immediately after protons in the slice have been excited by 90 degree pulse.

79)ac

A succession of 90 and 180 degree RF pulses ,each of different frequency, are used in multislice technique .Gap between slices is not needed to avoid cross- talk in this technique.

80) abe

In Spin echo, turbulent flow usually appear dark.Conventional T1 weighting with presaturation pulses produces dark blood flow.

81) ace

The image is obtained by applying inverse Fourier transform to k-space data. A component close to the center corresponds to a low spatial frequency oscillation.

82)abce

Signal in MR can be increased by decreasing the number of phase-encoding steps.

83)ab

Permanent magnet used in MRI cannot be shut down and produce only low field strength up to 0.3T.

84)ade

Faraday cage refers to wire mess incorporated in wall of the room. Faraday cage is used to screen the scanner from external (lift. power cables etc) RF interference.

85)ab

Angular momentum depicts the rotational motion of body. Angular momentum is vector in nature. Rotational angular momentum = angular velocity x moment of inertia.

86) ade

The gray matter and white matter

differ in water content by 10% only.TI time of gray matter and T1 of white matter (at 1T) differ by 1.5 .

87)ade

In inversion recovery pulse sequence, the rate at which −Mz returns toward +Mz depends on tissue T1 relaxation time. Magnitude of Mz is zero at time equal to 0.69T1.

88) ace

The image is obtained by applying inverse Fourier transform to k-space data. A component close to the center corresponds to a low spatial frequency oscillation.

89) bcd

Spin density images uses long TR and short TE. T2 weighted image use long TR to minimize T1 tissue differences.

90)abcd
91) abc

T1 cannot be measured directly. T1 is not always greater than T2. T1 can be nearly same as T2 or T1 can be larger than T2.

92) abc

T1 cannot be measured directly. T1 is not always greater than T2. T1 can be nearly same as T2 or T1 can be larger than T2.

93) bcde

Niobium-titanium is a semiconductor.

94)ace

Stimulated echoes as well as spin echoes contribute to the PSIF signal. It is useful in rapid acquisition of fluid sensitive images.
95)bde

Keyhole imaging acquires only the low spatial frequency information. TRICKS provides high- frame rate 3D images.
96)ce

In Time-0f-Flight MRA, there is suppression of background tissue signal and retention of signal from flowing blood. Intentional saturation of stationary tissues makes them appear dark.
97)ade

Regarding chemical shift, nucleus effectively shielded by electrons has high shielding constant. Higher is the shielding constant , lower is the resonance frequency.
98)abcde
99) bd

DC is used to generate magnetic field gradient. A narrow bandwidth of RF pulse contain a small range of frequencies. Only protons in a certain thin slice of patient is excited by the RF pulse.
100) abe

In multiecho technique, peak amplitudes of echo decrease with time constant T2. The first echo may produce PD weighted image.
`**101) ace**
Dark appearance of fast moving

blood on SE echo is because some of blood exited by 90 degree pulse has already left the slice before the 180 degree pulse occurs. In GRE scan, flowing blood and CSF usually appear bright .

102) abcde

SE sequence generally gives a bigger signal than GRE.

103)d

Resistive electromagnet is a set of DC coils with copper or aluminium conductors, consume some 5-100Kw of power. Heating limits its field strength to 0.5T. It produce vertical of horizontal field.

104)abe

Pregnant patient should not be exposed above 2.5T. Ethics committee approval required above 4T.

105)be

In spin echo sequence ,180 degree pulse is used to remove the H-field inhomogeneity. 90 degree pulse is followed by 180 degree pulse.

106)cde

Data in the central region has low frequency component. Data in the outer region has high frequency component.

107) acd

In phased-array coils individual coils are magnetically decoupled. Disadvantage of phased array coils are greater expense and longer reconstruction time.

108)ade

In permanent magnet ,the iron yoke and posts act as mechanical structure and flux return. The pole pieces shape B_O.

109)abcde
110)bce

Projection reconstruction acquisitions sample k-space on radial lines that pass through center of k-space and reduce motion artifact.

111)acde

In TOF ,repeated RF saturate stationary tissues and produce dim signal.

112)ade

The amplitude of the signal is not proportional to the concentration of the metabolite. Chemical shifts is independent of magnetic field strength.

113)ade

Larmor frequency is proportional to product of of magnetic field strength and gyromagnetic ratio.

114) ad

Small, lightweight molecules with little inertia(water, urine ,csf. Amniotic fluid) and atoms in solids and rigid macromolecules (compact bone,teeth,calculi metallic teeth)has large T1.

115)abce

Fat appear extremely bright on FSE T2-weighted image.

116)ade

No Contrast is required in GRE.

For good three dimensional(volume) angiography with high signal to noise , high velocity flow is needed.

117) abde

Noise can reduced by having larger gaps between slice.

118)ce

Resistive electromagnet has significant fringe fields and its ramp –up time is 15-30min.

119)abcde

120)ade

The lowest energy state of two interacting electron is when the spin angular momentum is in anti parallel direction. The configuration of lowest energy states between electron is usually called spin pairing.

121) de

FID is in form of amplitude versus time. Fourier transformation of FID is in form of frequency versus time .Shape of FT of FID is symmetrical about the Larmor frequency.

122) ace

Noise limits the visibility of low contrast structures.Image averaging improves SNR.

123)bcde

Defining line for safety purpose in MRI is 5G-line.

124) abce

Magnet made of neodymium-iron-boron has high temperature sensitivity.

125)abc

Fat appear intense on TSE . TSE produce higher SAR.

126)ade

In spiral scanning ,the spiral trajectory begins at center of k-space and are less susceptible to flow artifact than other rapid imaging technique.

127) ad

In TOF,distal flow is better retained with smaller flip angle. Placing the imaging slice in the plane of the vessel(in-plane saturation) is undesirable. Small voxel is often used to better visualize small vessels.

128)abe

The major metabolites in a ^{1}H spectrum cover a range of about 10ppm. Chemical shift dispersion plays major role in volume selection and in acquisition technique.

129)de

Gyromagnetic ratio of nucleus is a constant property of nucleus. In the quantum theory, a frequency of 42.6MHz corresponds to a quantum energy of 0.2micro ev.Antiparallel state of proton has 0.2micro eV lower energy than parallel state.

130)abce

Much of dephasing effect in T2 decay is due to field inhomogeneities due to machine factor.

131)abd

FSE is incompatible with respiratory compensation technique. Smaller voxel improve spatial resolution.

132)abd

Perfusion imaging uses paramagnetic contrast and usually need EPI.

133)abe

STIR sequence is used to suppress signal from fat.T2 weighting specifically increases contrast between normal and abnormal tissues.

134)abcde

135)ae

Nucleons posses orbital angular momentum. Protons and neutrons have the same spin and therefore same spin angular momentum. There are energy levels for the nucleons.

136) abcde

137)acd

Two pulses are separated by time TE/2. Muscle,tendon,liver appear dark on T2- imaging.

138) abcde

139)abcd

Superconducting magnet needs low electrical power.

140)abc

TSE may give false impression of being T1 weighted.TSE is relatively insensitive to susceptibility effects of blood products.

141)ace

Null point of tissue is given by 0.69X T1.The resonance frequency separation between fat and water signal increases at higher magnetic field.

142)acde

InTOF, Bright fat signal is a problem.

143)abcde

144)abd

After 3T2 ,only 5%of maximum signal remain. Greater the proportion of free water in the tissue,longer is T2.

145)bcd

Initial 180 degree pulse in inversion technique is used to accentuate T1 weighting. The tissue with longer T1 is suppressed.

146)d

Gd DTPA is water-insoluble,doesnot cross blood-brain barrier, increase contrast between pathological and normal tissue ,affect proton in water than that in fat.

147)acde

Gd, Mn, Fe are positive contrast agent.

148)ace

Superconducting magnet has significant fringe field. Weighs some 6 tones.

149)abd

Time –varying gradient fields are no symptoms below 20T/s. There appears to be no effect on fetal development.

150)bd

A proton pairs with themselves like neutrons.The nuclear spin is either zero or multiple of ½,or whole number. Charged nucleus is spinning and has angular momentum.

151)ade

In Fast SE (RARE or turboSE) relatively shorter TR is used than conventional SE. There is repeated application of 90 degree refocusing pulses.

152)abcde

153)bde

Superconducting magnet exihibit zero electrical resistance below critical temperature.Type II superconductors maintain superconductivity in high magnetic field.

154)abcde

155)cde

The resonance frequency of fat is slightly higher than that of water protons.Fat and water magnetization are in phase for echo times of 4.6msec,9.6msec etc at 1.5T.

156)acd

In TOF,3D TOF has better spatial resolution than 2D TOF. Gradually increasing flip angle is used in TONE

157)abde

In ^{1}H-MR spectroscopy, Choline— 3.2 ppm 16)abcd

Presence of grating lobes is an disadvantage.It reduce contrast resolution.

158)acde

Mxy is perpendicular to B .

159)de

Causes of T2 dephasing are machine factor and tiny additional field(around 1microT) produced by each neighbouring proton. Local variation in magnetic field is greatest in solids and rigid micomolecules and least in free water, amniotic fluid,and csf.

160)bd

Inversion recovery sequence produce T1-weighted image. TR used is about 3T1 to ensure nearly total recovery between pulse.It gives good grey –white discrimination.

161)bcd

Gadolinium are has seven unpaired electron is contraindicated in renal failure .

162) abce

Areas of uptake of supra paramagnetic agents appear black.

163)cd

In superconducting electromagnet , it takes several

hours for the coil to cool down and the current to build up. The coil is then short circuited and the power is never removed. Some 200kWh energy remains stored within the superconducting coil.

164)bcd

Acoustic noise in MR increases with higher gradient amplitudes and higher field strength in GRE.There is possibility of hearing damage to fetus.

165)acd

For the loop of wire , larger the electron flow , the more quickly the loop align in the magnetic field. The MDM of L shell electron is equal to two Bohr Magneton.

166)bce

In superconducting magnet, the entire magnetic system must be maintained at about 4 degree K. Liquefied helium gas has very low boiling point.

167)abcde

168)bce

In Fast SE fat appears brighter than conventional SE due to reduction in j-coupling effect. There is less susceptibility effect, so disadvantageous for detecting hemorrhage.

169)abcde
170)de

Superconducting wire used in MRI is embedded in copper matrix. The copper is the primary current conduction pathway above the critical temperature of the superconducting wire. The cupper stabilizer significantly reduces a magnet s propensity to quench.

171) abe

TurboSTIR has more contrast and less blurring than its TSE.

172)cde

T2 of the free water pool is longer than that of the bound water pool. The width in frequency of the resonance of the free pool is smaller than that of the bound pool.

173)acd

2D TOF is compatible with breath holding. 3D TOF provide better spatial resolution than 2D TOF.

174)abcde
175)d

Compact bone and tendon, Teeth and calculi, metallic clip ,Fat has short T2

176) acd

Anti parallel spins recover more quickly in fat than water. T1 of water is longer than fat .

177) ce

Gd-DTPA are water- soluble., shorten both T1 and T2 , but effect is more on T1,T1 weighting is used after gadolinium injection.

178) bcde

Xenon dissolves in blood.

179)abcd

Care must be taken when replenishing the cryogen. Air entering the system would solidify like a plug.

180) be

Specific absorption ratio(SAR) is the RF energy deposited per mass of tissue expressed as Watts/Kilogram. Skin and rectal temperature should not exceed 1degree Celsius. SAR is greater for large body parts.

181) abcde

182) abcde

183)bcde

Surface coils are used as receiver only.

184)abcd

There is more RF deposition in magnetization transfer.

185)abd

With low bandwidth, smaller FOV is used. Low bandwidth produce greater chemical –shift artifact.

186)abe

In active shielding, a secondary coil carry current in the opposite direction as the main coil. The field stability in superconducting MRI is not governed by power supply .**187)abde**

No RF spoiling is implemented in SSFP.

188)abcde

189) abc

Permanent magnet used in MRI is expensive to buy but the cheapest to run and requires no power to run.

190)acd

During relaxation, Mxy decreases and Mz increases. As Mz increases, strength of MR signal decreases.

191)ade

T1 value increases with magnetic field strength. T2 value remains more or less unaffected with magnetic field strength.

192)abd

193)abd

Gd-DTPA is positive contrast agent.

194) bcde

Spatial resolution is increased by reducing in pixel size and FOV.

195) abcde

196) abcd197)acde

One Tesla=10^4 Gauss.

198)abcde

199)bce

FLASH – Fast low angle shot, FAST- Fourier acquired steady state technique

200)abde

Chemical artifact is produced in the frequency encoding direction.

201) bcde

In inversion recovery sequence 180 degree pulse invert magnetization fro +z axis to -z axis .

202)abe

T1 weighted images are less degraded by crosstalk than T2weighted images, so that the slice gap of 10 to 30% may be adequate. Cross talk may be reduced by the use of longer RF.

203)cde

SSFP does not show saturation effect and is motion insensitive.

204)abcde

205)abcde

206)abcd

T1 of tissue lengthens in the stronger magnetic field. FID decays with time constant of $T2^*$ of a few milliseconds. Static magnetic field is not perfectly uniform.

207.

Gd cause susceptibility effect in perfused tissues. The tracer concentration is roughly proportional to the relaxation rate in normally perfused tissues.

208)ace

Reducing number of encodings reduce scan time. Short scan time reduce motion artefacts.

209)ab

Magnetic field used in MRI must be uniform to 5 ppm over a large volume for imaging(1 ppm for spectroscopy).Magnetic field Is usually aligned vertically in permanent magnet.

210)abcde

211)bde

The MDM of nuclei are not calculated, they are measured for each nucleus.MDM of the nuclei cannot be calculated by adding

neutrons in the nucleus.

212)cde

Mxyprecess around the main magnetic field at Larmor frequency .Only Mxy can be detected, the regrowth of M_Z cannot be detected.

213)ae

Residual Mz is proportional to the cosine of the flip angle. No 180 degree pulse is used. During negative readout gradient, there is dephasing of spins.

214)abe

STIR produce fat suppression independent of Bo homogeneity. Tissue with longer T1 (gray matter ,csf) appear brighter than tissues with shorter T1(white matter, fat).

215)abcde

216)abcde

217)abcde

218)cde

In fast spin- echo ,scan time=TR x Number of phase encoded lines x number of excitations/ETL.FSE increases RF deposition.

219)abcde

220)abce

PC utilizes the phase information to obtain MR angiogram, images of directional flow, and flow quantification.

221)bde

Mz recovers during spin lattice relaxation. After three time constants (3T1) ,recovery is 95% complete.

222.abcde--
223)abc
224)abe
The greater the tip angle, the greater the T1 weighting. For T2 and PD weighting, use 5--10 degree of tip angle.
225.abd
High tesla MR cause an increase in tissue T1s (prolonged blood signal and better background suppression for time-of-flight angiography) and increased chemical shift artifact
226)abcde
227) ade
In spin- labeled image ,blood-water magnetization is in different state from that of tissue-water magnetization. In controlled image blood- water magnetization – is in same state from that of tissue-water magnetization.
228)ade
Wrap-round of image occurs in phase encoding direction. Electronic circuit are designed to suppress aliasing in frequency encoding direction.
229) ad
The fringe field of a permanent magnet is negligible as it is concentrated within the iron yoke.Stronger is the magnetic field, stronger is the fringe field. Shimming coil reduce fringe field.
230) abcde
131) abcd
Nuclear spin of ^{14}N is one(1).
232)ade
The frequency of the RF pulse selects the location of slice .The bandwidth of the RF pulse selects the thickness of slice.

233)abcd
Felix and Purcell shared the Nobel Prize for physics in 1952.
234) abe
STIR cannot distinguish fat from blood products.STIR paradoxically reduce signal in contrast enhanced setting.
235)abe
Changing the matrix size along the frequency-encoding direction has no effect on scan time.Decrease in matrix size exacerbates truncation artifact.
236.abcde
237)be
Gradient amplitude defines the maximum field strength of a gradient system(millitesla/meter).
Gradient duty cycle describes the percentage of time gradient subsystem can provide maximum gradient strength pulse sequence waveforms.
X and Y gradient coils(saddle-shaped) has different geometry than the Z gradient(cylindrical).
238)ade

Incoherent GRE ,the spoiler gradient disperses any residual transverse magnetization that remains after the signal has been read. The flip angle that produces the most signal for the given TR and T1 is known as the Ernst angle.
239)abd
The effect of MRI contrast agent is observed indirectly. The diagnostic potential of paramagnetic agents was first demonstrated in patients by Young, using ferric chloride.
240) bc

In PC angiography phase shift is proportional to the velocity of blood flow .Choose a velocity encoding range (V_{ENC}) that is slightly higher than the maximal anticipated velocity in the vessel of interest. Velocity aliasing shows abrupt transition of phase in the vessel.

241 abcde

242)abcd

T1 and T2 of water is approximately 3000ms.

243)abc

Dephasing of Mxy starts immediately after 90 degree pulse. Rephasing starts just after 180 degree pulse.

244)abd

The positive gradient pulse(x) duration is twice that of the negative gradient pulse(x^1).Moving blood appears bright.

245)abcde

246)abd

Sensitivity weighting factor in diffusion imaging depend the time and the amplitude of the diffusion gradient. Signal attenuation is directly related to the apparent(or effective) diffusion coefficient multiplied by sensitivity weighting factor.

247)abde

Motion artefacts in MRI are usually apparent in the phase encoding direction.

248)abcde

249) abcde

250)abde

Nuclear spin of ^{23} Na. is 3/2.

251)abd

Slice crosstalk is due to fact that RF pulse is not precise in frequency. Slice crosstalk degrade the image quality, so it is common to leave a gap between slices in MRI.

252)abcde

253)abcde

254)ae

Imaging at 3T produce superior fat suppression, more chemical shift and more power deposition.

255)bcde

The coil used to produce linear fields (B_1) is known as linear transmit coils. The quadrature transmit coils produce circular B_1 field

256)bde

In steady-state free precession GRE there is recycling of transverse magnetization that persist after readout to increase the signal intensity of certain tissues. The difference in contrast behavior between spoiled and SSFP GRE is manifested only conditions of TR</-T2 and large flip angle.

257)d

Diamagnetic substance has no net electron spin. Paramagnetic has net electron spin. Paramagnetic substance has odd number of electron. Gd has seven unpaired electron.

258)abe

Regarding display in PC angiography speed image is ideal for anatomic depiction of vascular anatomy. There is no information regarding flow direction in speed image the complex difference image.

259)bce

T1 of Fat is approximately 250ms in field of 1T Bone and teeth very long T1 and very short T2.

260)abcde

261)abcde

262)abcd

Magnetic susceptibility effect of GRE is useful in detection of hemorrhagic lesion.

263)ce

In DWI, gradient pulses are applied after RF excitation. Gradients used must be strong. Tissues with normal random thermal motion/diffusion attenuates due to destructive interference of all the phase-dispersed spins.

64)abde

The faster the motion, more spacing of the ghost images occur.

265) abcde

266)abcde

267) de

The nucleus cannot come in exact alignment with the magnetic field. The up orientation has slightly lower energy than that of down orientation. Very few nuclei of tissue participate in the NMR signal.

268) acde

At the end of phase encoding, all Mxy vectors are precessing at the same rate but not all M_{XY} vectors are in the same phase.

269)abd

Protons and neutrons possess magnetic dipole moment that is proportional to their intrinsic spin. Spin of ^{23}Na is 3/2.

270)abcde

271) abe

Fat and water is in phase when TE is in even multiple of 3.4ms.Fat water signal modulation does not occur in SE sequence.

272)bcd

^{16}O,^{14}N,^{12}C possess no nuclear magnetism. ^{31}P has lower gyromagnetic ratio(17.2MHz) than that of ^{1}H. Magnetic field should be uniform to better than 1ppm.

273)acd

In balanced coherent gradient echo bile, blood and csf,fat appear bright and there is tendency to have dark stripes in the image.

274)abcde

275)abcde

276)ade

Correct order of T1 value is fat< Liver<white matter and Grey matter<CSF<water.

277)ade

The slice thickness is reduced by decreasing the RF bandwidth or by increasing the gradient of the magnetic field. Thinner slice produce less partial volume effect.

278)acd

TI weighting is possible in echo planar imaging. There may problem of artifact.

279)cd

Oxyhaemoglobin is diamagnetic while deoxyhaemoglobin is paramagnetic. During activity , deoxyhaemoglobin increase.

280) abc

MRI with high field is more hazardous to patient and produce more chemical artifact.

281)abcde

282) abcde

283) acde

Slice select gradient is removed at

the end of 90 degree pulse.

284)ade

Frequency of precession= gyromagnetic ratio x applied field strength. When spin system is in thermal equilibrium, slightly more spins are in the lower energy state.

285) bce

With incoherent GRE,transverse magnetization after signal readout is dispersed.

Transverse magnetization is refocused and reutilized after readout in coherent GRE.

286)ab

In magnetization transfer off resonance MT RF pulses saturates the restricted pool. Mobile pool becomes saturated due to exchange of magnetization between two pools. Here the signal from mobile protons decrease.

287) abde

In multislice imaging ,a new slice cannot be excited until the echo from the previous slice has been completely detected.

288) abd

1T is about 20000 times greater than the earth's magnetic field. Patient become slightly magnetized inside the coil.

289)abcd

In EPI typical scan time 50-200micosecond. There is no ghost images due to breathing and cardiac pulsation seen.

290)de

Diamagnetic always align ant parallel to external field. Paramagnetic align parallel to external magnetic field. Ferromagnetic material possess magnetism outside the magnetic field.

291)cde

In PCA,image intensity is related to phase ,it is reflection of blood motion along a gradient rather than inflow into the slice.

292)bcde

TR and TE are both short in T1W image.

293)abce

The number of lines filled in the k space matches the number of encodings in the sequence.

294)cde

Resolution ,echo strength, and signal to noise ratio are compromised in echo planar imaging. The strong magnetic field is necessary.

295)abcd

296) abe

Magnetic susceptibility may lead to increase or decrease in MR signal

297)bce

Shim coil and gradient coil carry DC current. Steeper the slice –select gradient , the thinner the slice.

298) abcde

299) abce

Larmor frequency of $^{31}P= 17.24$ MHz/T.

300) bcd

In spin echo sequence the time interval between each 90 degree is called the TR interval.Time for acquiring image in spin echo=phase encoding steps X TR x averages.

301)ade

Nutation refers to the spiraling movement of M toward the x-y plane. Excitation pulse refers to RF pulse used to convert longitudinal magnetization into transverse magnetization.

302)abe

Balanced steady state free precession,SSFP is insensitive to motion artifact. Fluid and fat appear bright.

303)cd

In MT contrast mobile protons resonate over narrow range of resonance frequencies. Restricted protons resonate over wide range of frequencies.MT pulses has minor effect on fat or that of Gd – enhanced tissue.

304)abde

STIR has not stringent requirement of static field homogeneity.

305)abe

Single-shot EPI eliminate any degree of T1 weighting and T2 weighting is improved .It is helpful in characterization of short T1, short T2 lesions such as cyst and hemangioma.

306) acde

Positive contrast agent dominantly lower T1 and increase signal.

307) abcd

PCA takes longer time than TOF.

308)bcd

TR and TE are both long in T2W image. Water and CSF appear brighter than fat on T2W image.

309)acd

The central part of k space contains data low spatial frequencies.

310)abcd

Generally speaking , the phase encoding gradient is best applied along the shorter dimension of the patient anatomy.

311) ace

For MRI to be feasible, a nuclide must high low gyromagnetic ratio. A high magnetic field(>2T) is needed to give sufficient signal strength and sufficiently good spatial resolution.

312)cd

Chemical shift artifact is noted in frequency –encoding direction .Fat has slightly higher resonant frequency in comparison to water. Stronger static field produces greater shift in terms of pixel.

313) bc

Increasing TR increases SNR and decreasing TR may increase T1 contrast.

314) bce

Spin up state has lower energy than the spin down state. The Larmor frequency of precession is exactly equal to frequency of radiation absorbed in a transition from one spin state to another.

CHAPTER 10
ULTRASOUND

1. True regarding transducer with high Q-value

a) has narrower bandwidth as transmitter

b) has narrower bandwidth as receiver

c) produce pure note

d) heavy damping

e) good for pulsed ultrasound

2.True regarding ultrasound contrast agents

a)Air-filled microspheres improve ventricular visualization diagnosis of DVT

b) Low- solubility gas encapsulated in a lipid wall is used in vascular application

c)Perfluorocarbonnanoprticles are used to improve imaging of peripheral vascular disease

d)Perfluorocarbon nanoparticles stay in blood transiently for seconds

e)Gold-bound colloidal microtubes may be immunologically targeted

3.True regarding pulsed Doppler

a)Sampling volume is positioned over the vessel of interest

b)Range gate is set to receive echoes only from selected sampling volume

c) A low PRF is chosen for superficial vessel

d) As range setting is increased, the PRF is increased

e) The depth of sampling volume determines the PRF needed

4.True regarding matching layer

a)It is used in front of transducer

b) Improve transmission of ultrasound from transducer to patient and not vice-versa

c) The thickness of matching layer must be equal to half of ultrasound wavelength in the matching layer

d)Impedance of matching layer must be similar to that of soft tissue

e)Made of mixture of aluminium powder and epoxy resin

5.True regarding backing block of transducer

a)Backing block is made of epoxy resin and suspended tungsten

b) Backing block results into long pulse

c)Backing block results into low Q-value

d) Sound output is increased if disc is backed by air

e) High Q-value results if disc is backed by air

6.Advantages of tissue harmonic imaging

a)Reduced reverberation artifact

b)Reduced distortion and scattering from fatty tissue

c)Improved contrast resolution

d)Better visualization of low contrast lesions and liquid filled cavities

e) Reduced acoustic noise

7.True regarding aliasing

a) Aliasing is consequence of sampling requirement

b)The PRF determines the minimum velocity that can be measured without aliasing

c)It is easy to measure fast flow in deep blood vessels

d)Aliasing can be reduced by use of lower frequency transducer and increasing the Doppler angle and PRF

e)Aliasing occurs in pulsed and continuous wave Doppler

8 True regarding ultrasound

a) Pulse rate and frequency are same

b)Duration of sonic pulse varies with Q-factor

c) The pulse rate determines the total number of echoes returning to the transducer in a unit of time

d)As the pulse rate increases, the receiving time increases

e) At pulse rate of 10000, the thickest part that can be examined is 75cm

9.True regarding ultrasound

a) Bandwidth is the full width at half-maximum intensity of the frequency spectrum

b) Nearly parallel part of ultrasound beam is known as Fraunhofer region

c) Side lobes refers to small beams of low intensity ultrasound outside the beam

d) The thickness of tissue that reduces the sound intensity to half its original value is called it's the half-value layer

e)Dynamic range of any component of an ultrasound imager is the ratio of the maximum intensity of the signal to the minimum intensity that can be detected

10.True regarding harmonic imaging

a)First harmonic used to form image

b) Filtering and pulse inversion are used to isolate second harmonic

c)Pulse inversion degrades axial resolution

d) Motion artifact may occur with pulse inversion

e)In pulse inversion ,every other pulse polarity is reversed

11.True regarding real-time color flow imaging

a) use color code to show the direction and velocity of flow

b)the depth of each color varies with the velocity of flow

c) longer pulse is used as compared to normal B-scan

d)Estimate only the mean velocity and variance of velocity

e) Aliasing is not feature of color scan

12.True regarding ultrasound

a)Focused transducer decreases lateral resolution

b) The lens material used in focusing is usually polystyrene or epoxy resin

c) The ultrasound is maximally restricted and of greatest intensity at focal poin

d) A close approximation of the focal length is diameter of the lens

e) Focusing moves the transition zone towards the lens

13.True regarding ultrasound

a)4-D imaging refers to the acquisition and display of volume images in real time.

b) Micrbubbles are used for reperfusion imaging.

c)Digital scan converter is used to enable freeze frame.

d)Tran vascular transducer is used to assess stents.

e)Percentage of ultrasound reflected by bone –muscle is 30%.

14.True regarding power Doppler

a)Map the amplitude of the Doppler signal.

b)Emphasize the quantity of blood flow.

c) The color indicates velocity or flow direction.

d) Less dependent on insonation angle.

e) weaker signals cannot be imaged than in color image.

15. True regarding ultrasound

a) Ultrasound encountering RBCs are scattered in one direction ,referred to as Rayleigh –Tyndall scattering.

b)Factor two(2) in Doppler shift equation is due to double Doppler shift.

c)Wave length of 3.5MHz transducer is 0.44mm.

d)The intensity of scattered ultrasound wave in Rayleigh-Tyndall scattering decreases with the fourth power of the frequency.

e)Doppler shift falls within the audible range of frequency.

16.True regarding ultrasound

a)Broad bandwidth reduce speckle.

b)There is no need of compression and remapping of backscattered signal.

c)A-mode displays echo amplitude and the position of moving reflectors.

d)Electronic beam steering is used in linear array and phased array transducer.

e)Linear array transducer is commonly used in vascular application.

17.True regarding focusing

a) Focusing produces stronger echoes.

b) Focusing decreases the lateral resolution.

c) The shorter the focal length, the narrower and shorter the focal region.

d) Shorter focal length produce less divergence of beam.

e)The greater the curvature, the shorter the focal length.

18.True regarding axial or depth resolution

a) Axial resolution is the ability to separate two interfaces.

b) The axial resolution is about twice the pulse length.

c) the higher the frequency of ultrasound, the better the axial resolution.

d) the longer the pulse length, the better the axial resolution.

e) The axial resolution improves by omitting backing block.

19.True regarding power Doppler

a)The amplitude of signal depend on the number of RBCs.

b) Differentiate areas of flow and no flow.

c)Not useful for imaging smaller vessels.

d) Aliasing noted.

e) tissue motion creates artefacts.

20.True regarding continuous wave Doppler transducer

a)Use of single piezoelectric elements.

b) Use of low Q-factor transducer.

c) Use of transducer with air as backing material.

d) No quarter wave matching needed.

e) Inclined transducer elements.

21.Methods of focusing are

a) Concave piezoelectric element.

b) Spherical piezoelectric element.

c)Plastic acoustic (concave or convex) lens.

d)Curved mirror.

e)Electronic focusing.

22.True regarding quality assurance of ultrasound machine

a) Resolution tested by imaging a test rig.

b)sensitivity, dynamic range tested by Perspex block test.

c)Grey scale performance and Doppler function tested by tissue mimicking phantom.

d) Power output of transducer measured by force balance.

e) power output of transducer measured by calorimeter.

23.True regarding higher frequency ultrasound

a) Less attenuation by soft tissue.

b) Produce stronger scattered signal.

c) Can be more sharply defined.

d) Causes larger Doppler shift.

e)Used for deeper structures.

24. True regarding acoustic impedance

a) Practically independent of frequency of transducer.

b) The greater the difference in acoustic impedance, the lesser the fraction of sound energy reflected.

c) The transducer and backing block need no matching of acoustic impedance.

d) Acoustic impedance of matching plate should be intermediate between transducer and skin.

e)Does not depend upon elasticity of material.

25.-10MHz transducer is used for

a)The thyroid.

b)The carotid.

c)The breast.

d)Infants.

e) Eye.

26.True regarding ultrasound

a)The intensity of an ultrasound beam is least in the focal region.

b) The time –averaged intensity may exceed 100 Mw/cm^2.

c) The total sound energy should nowhere exceed 50J/cm^2.

d) Local heating effect of ultrasound is used therapeutically.

e) May cause mechanical damage to

cell membranes.

27. True regarding Doppler

a) CW Doppler is very sensitive to weak signals.
b) CW Doppler provides depth information.
c) CW Doppler is used to monitor fetal heart sounds.
d) Pulsed Doppler provides depth as well as velocity information.
e) Gating is used in CW Doppler.

28. True regarding levovist

a) Mixture comprising 9.1% microcrystalline galactose micro particles and 99.9% palmitic acid.
b) Doesnot traverse the pulmonary bed.
c) Bubble diameter –approximately 2 micrometer.
d)Enhance color and spectral Doppler signals
e)Enhance gray scale exam using nonlinear imaging modes

29. True regarding effect of acoustic impedance attention

a) Gas filled organ cast shadow.
b) Partial reflection of sound energy occurs at any interface with air or gas.
c) Coupling gel is used to avoid trapping of air between transducer and skin.
d)Reflection less than .01% are unlikely to be detected.
e)Normal lung cannot be penetrated.

30. True regarding cavitations

a) Cause chemical damage to cellular constituents.

b) More likely to occur at high pressures and low frequencies.
c)More likely to occur with pulse beams.
d) Micro bubbles expansion in a liquid or near liquid medium.
e)Enormous rise of temperature on collapse of micro bubbles.

31. True regarding ultrasound

a)Ultrasound requires 13 microsecond for a round trip of 1cm.
b) The required time between successive pulses is at least 26 microsecond per cm of range in the sample volume.
c) The maximum Doppler shift frequency that can be detected by a pulsed Doppler system is equal to twice the pulse repetition frequency(PRF).
d) PRF determines the depth at which a Doppler shift signal can be detected.
e) PRF determines the minimum Doppler shift that can be detected without encountering aliasing.

32. Correct matching of acoustic impedance($kg/m^2/s$)

a)Muscle 1.38×10^6
b)Liver 1.64×10^6
c)Spleen 1.63×10^6
d)kidney 1.62×10^6
e)Fat 1.70×10^6

33. True regarding Doppler effect

a)Higher the transducer frequency, the greater the Doppler frequency shift.
b)The faster the interface moves,

the greater the Doppler frequency shift.

c) The maximum Doppler shift frequency is obtained when the angle of insonation is 90 degree.

d) The Doppler frequency shift is comparatively large .

e) The Doppler shift frequency shift is equivalent to an audio frequency(0-10KHz).

34.True regarding ultrasound

a)Thermal index= the power emitted/the power required to increase the temperature by 1degree Celsius.

b)The thermal index is an indication of temperature rise in the tissue.

c) The mechanical index= the peak rarefaction pressure/the square root of the ultrasound frequency.

d) The mechanical index is a measure of the maximum amplitude of the pressure pulse.

e)The mechanical index value less than 0.5 are below the threshold level of any effect.

35.Ultrasound is subject to

a)Reflection.
b)Refraction.
c)Diffraction.
d)Scattering.
e)Absorption.

36.True regarding ultrasound contrast agents

a)Enhance echo by increasing backscatter of the tissue.

b)Second generation agent use air.

c)Colloidal suspensions of liquids such as perfluorocarbons are taken up by reticuloendothelial system.

d)Levovist provide enhancement in the parenchyma of the liver and spleen.

e) Useful imaging time while using levovist and echovist is much more then minutes.

37.True regarding artefacts

a)Speckle artifact gives textured appearance to liver, spleen etc.

b)Reverberation artifact produce series of delayed echoes equally spaced in time.

c)The structures in liver may appear in lung due to reverberation.

d) Negative shadow is due to acoustic shadowing.

e)Ring down is due to gas bubbles.

38.True regarding phased array scanners

a) Each element is less than half wavelength wide.

b)Unlike a linear array ,all the elements are used to generate each beam in the sweep.

c)The transmission focus and reception foci lie on angled scan lines.

d)Like linear array and annular array probes,variableaperture,apodization and focusing are possible in both transmission and reception.

e) Advantage over mechanical sector scanner is their ability to perform mixed mode scanning.

39.True regarding ultrasound

a. In most diagnostic applications,

frequencies in the 2–20MHz (wavelength of 1 to 0.1mm)range are used

b. capacitative microfabricated ultrasound transducers (CMUTs) is based on photo etching

c. 1 or 2MHz transducers is used for the abdomen in obese subjects, and for transcranial studies

d. For average soft tissues, the ultrasound loss amounts to approximately 1dB per cm tissue depth for each MHz.

e. Frequencies as high as 20MHz can be used for imaging the eye and skin, and for intravascular ultrasound (IVUS)

40.True regarding specular reflectors

a) Small and smooth interface.
b)Diaphragm.
c)Wall of urine filled bladder.
d)Endometrial stripe.
e)Angle of insonation independent.

41.True regarding ultrasound

a)Frequency>20kMz.
b) Inaudible to humans.
c) Narrow beam as well as light.
d)Electromagnetic radiation.
e)Undergoes reflection and refraction.

42. True regarding ultrasound

a) The thickness of matching plate is a quarter of a wavelength.
b)Roughly penetration of ultrasound (cm) = 40 /frequency (MHz)

c)Vascular transducer operate at 10-20MHz.
d) Frame rate x lines per frame = PRF.
e) Depth of view=0.5 x sound velocity / PRF.

43.True regarding ultrasound transducer

a)Convert electrical energy into ultrasonic energy and vice versa.
b) medical crystal is made to vibrate in radial mode.
c) Quartz is man-made material which possess piezoelectric properties.
d) Barium titanate was the first of the ceramic ferroelectrics to be discovered.
e)Lead zirconatetitanate (PZT) is used as piezoelectric material in the transducer.

44.True regarding speed of ultrasound

a) The mean value of speed of ultrasound in soft tissue is 1540m/s.
b)Speed decreases with increase in temperature.
c)Acoustic impedance depend on frequency of ultrasound.
d)Acoustic impedance of tissues differ from each other by high percentage.
e) Rayl is unit of acoustic impedance.

45.True regarding transducer

a) convert electrical signal into ultrasound wave.
b)Piezo-ceramic disc made of lead

zirconatetitanate (PZT).

c)Piezo-ceramic disc made of polyvinylidinedifluoride (PVDF).

d) May be autoclaved.

e)Silver coating on both side of disc.

46.**True statements are**

a)Specular reflection(mirror) occurs when beam strikes a large smooth interface.

b)Diffuse reflection occurs when tissue interface is rough and has undulations equal to a wavelength or so.

c) Scattering occurs when sound encounters the structures much larger than wavelength.

d) Scattering follows Snell's rule.

e)Scattering allows even smaller structures to be visualized.

47.**True regarding transducer**

a) The Curie temperature is the temperature at which polarization of piezoelectric crystal is lost.

b) The Curie temperature of PZT-5A is about 365 degree Celsius.

c) The natural frequency is one that produces internal wavelength that are half the thickness of the crystal.

d)The frequency that correspond to twice of the wavelength thickness is called fundamental resonance frequency.

e) Crystal designed to resonate at high megahertz frequencies is extremely thin.

48. **True regarding ultrasound**

a)The instantaneous intensity at any point is related as P^2/Z (p—pressure ,z—acoustic impedance).

b)Spatial peak temporal intensity produced by machine depend on only the machine control.

c) The temporal average intensity help to determine temperature rise in sound absorbing medium.

d)Pulse bandwidth increases as pulse length increase.

e) A continuous wave has infinitely narrow bandwidth.

49.**True regarding contrast**

a)Bubbles respond asymmetrically to high intensity pressures and produce harmonics in the scattered waves.

b) The harmonic response of a ultrasound contrast depend on only incident pressure of ultrasound field.

c) In harmonic mode ,the system is tuned to receive echoes preferentially at double to that of transmit frequency.

d) Echoes from solid tissue as well as red blood cells are suppressed in harmonic mode.

e)Thump artifact due to clutter is completely absent in Doppler harmonic imaging.

50.**True regarding ultrasound**

a) Requires material medium to travel.

b) Transverse in nature.

c) Cannot be focused.

d) Does not undergo interference and diffraction.

e) Undergo reflection and

refraction.

51. True regarding attenuation of ultrasound

a) Absorption, scattering and partial reflection cause attenuation of ultrasound.
b) Higher the frequency of ultrasound, the lesser the attenuation.
c) Attenuation is usually measured in decibels.
d) Higher the frequency of transducer, the less the effective penetration power of the beam.
e) There is high absorption or scatter of ultrasound in water.

52. True regarding transducer

a) For polarization of piezoelectric crystal , the ceramic is heated to very high temperature in a strong electric field.
b) The transducer may be autoclaved.
c) The thickness of crystal determine its resonant frequency.
d) A frequency need transducer change.
e) Crystal need to be thin for high frequency probe.

53. Causes of ultrasound attenuation are

a) Divergence of sound beam.
b) Partial reflection at tissue interface.
c) Refraction at tissue interface.
d) Absorption in tissue.
e) Scattering in tissue.

54. True regarding tissue harmonic imaging

a) The tissue harmonic reduce contrast between the bubble and tissue rendering the problem of detecting perfusion more difficult.
b) The tissue is completely dark in a typical tissue harmonic image.
c) Reverberations are exaggerated by using tissue harmonic imaging.
d) Tissue harmonic imaging suppresses side lobe and other low level interference.
e) Routine USG modality of choice for visualizing solid structures.

55. True regarding velocity of ultrasound

a) The greater the density, lower the velocity.
b) The greater the compressibility, higher the velocity.
c) The smaller the elastic modulus, Greater the velocity.
d) Velocity is constant for given material.
e) Velocity depend upon temperature.

56. True regarding A-mode scan

a) Sometimes used for examining the eye.
b) The simplest form of ultrasound imaging.
c) Shows only position of tissue interfaces.
d) The location of the blip indicate

the depths of the corresponding interfaces along the beam.

e) The blip height is proportional to the echo strength.

57. True regarding high Q-transducer

a) Produce a nearly pure sound.

b) Produce sound covering much wider range of frequencies.

c) More efficient transmitter.

d) More useful for sonic imaging than Doppler.

e) has short ringing down time.

58. True regarding ultrasound

a) Attenuation coefficient refers to the rate of decrease of intensity with distance.

b) For most soft tissue , attenuation coefficient / frequency is a constant.

c) Edge effect artifact is due to scattering.

d) In Rayleigh scattering , scattering structures are much larger than a wavelength.

e) Coupling gel is used to reduce attenuation coefficient.

59. Unlike x-ray and gamma rays, ultrasound undergoes

a) Refraction.

b) Reflection.

c) Focusing.

d) Interference.

e) Diffraction.

60. True regarding ultrasound

a) Echoes equalized electronically by time gain compensation .

b) The transducer are pulsed at regular interval in A-mode and B-mode.

c) In B-mode ,returning echoes are displayed as vertical blip.

d) Real- time imaging demonstrate the motion of tissues.

e) Time gain is varied typically from 0 to 50 Db.

61. True regarding transducer

a) Q-factor refers to purity of sound.

b) Q-factor refers to the ring down time.

c) Q-factor=resonance frequency/frequency above resonance at which intensity is reduced by half-- frequency below resonance at which intensity is reduced by half.

d) Q-factor can be altered by changing characteristic of backing block.

e) Q –factor of PZT-5A is approximately 75.

62. True regarding ultrasound

a) Velocity of ultrasound in average soft tissue is 1540m/s.

b) Ultrasound takes nearly 70 microsecond to travel each centimeter in average soft tissue.

c) The wavelength of ultrasound (produced by transducer of 3.5MHz) in soft tissue is 0.9mm.

d) In typical diagnostic application, the particles travel to and fro through distances less than

1micrometere.

e)Velocity of ultrasound in typical bone is 3200m/s.

63.True regarding linear scan over sector scan

a)Needs larger area of patient contact.
b) Gives a better quality image .
c) Wider field of view near the skin.
d) Used in intracvitary probes.
e) Used to image heart.

64. Effects of cavitations are

a) Heat generation.
b) Free radical generation.
c) Microstreaming of fluid around the bubble.
d) Radiation forces.
e) Mechanical actions resulting from bubble collapse.

65.True regarding backing block

a)The backing block is incorporated to quench the vibrations and increase sonic pulse.
c) The ratio of tungsten to resin determine the impedance of backing block.
c) The rubber powder is used in backing block to increase the attenuation of sound in the backing block.
d)Impedance of backing block material differs widely from that of the transducer crystal.
e) Backing block does not affect Q-factor.

66.True regarding ultrasound

a)Higher the frequency ,shorter the near field.
b) Higher the frequency ,the less the beam divergence in far field.
c) Low frequency unfocussed beams are better collimated than high frequency ones.
d) Focusing produce narrower beam in the focal zone with increasing its intensity.
e) Focusing improves lateral resolution and sensitivity in focal zone.

67.True relationship is

a) Velocity = wavelength x frequency.
b) Acoustic impedance =density x velocity.
c)Intensity of ultrasound is proportional to the square of the wave amplitude.
d)Mechanical coefficient = mean frequency/ bandwidth.
e)In Doppler study, the change of frequency is proportional to the velocity of the interface

68.True regarding sector scan(mechanical versus electronic)

a)Mechanical sector scanner is generally cheap.
b) Electronic sector scanner has no moving parts.
c) Electronic sector transducer employs circular transducer.
d)Electronic sector transducer is more compact.
e) Transducer in mechanical sector

scanner moves within fluid filled plastic dome.

69. True regarding ultrasound

a) High frequency beam produce superior depth resolution.
b) High frequency beam produce shorter Fresnel zone.
c)Tissue absorption increases with increasing frequency.
d) High frequency beam is used for deeper structures.
e) Focusing partially overcome drawback of larger transducer.

70.True regarding ultrasound

a)Higher the frequency ,shorter the near field.
b) Higher the frequency ,the less the beam divergence in far field.
c) Low frequency unfocussed beams are better collimated than high frequency ones.
d) Focusing produce narrower beam in the focal zone with increasing its intensity.
e) Focusing improves lateral resolution and sensitivity in focal zone.

71.True regarding natural or resonant frequency of transducer

a) Produce a wavelength equal to the thickness of the piezoelectric disc.
b) The thicker the transducer , the lower the natural frequency.
c) Resonant frequency does not depend on material of transducer.
d) Transducer is most efficient as

transmitter and most sensitive as receiver at resonant frequency,
e)A 3.5MHz transducer has a disc about 0.5mm disc.

72.True regarding acoustic impedance

a) It is a constant for a particular substance.
b)Cgs unit is Rayl.
c) Greater the difference of impedance between two tissue, greater is the reflection.
d)Acoustic impedance of bone is $7.8x\ 10^{-5}$rayl.
e) Acoustic impedance of air is 0.0004×10^{-5}Rayl.

73.True regarding sensitivity

a) Sensitivity is measure of the weakest scatterer or reflector that can be distinguished from noise.
b)Sensitivity is poorest   close to transit focus.
c)Sensitivity depend on the focus position only.
d)The dynamic range of scanner is fixed. F
e)The dynamic range of scanner is measure of the minimum sensitivity that a scanner can achieve.

74.True regarding physical effect of ultrasound

a) Thermal effect is principally due to absorption.
b) Acoustically induced flow of fluid is known as streaming.
c) Acoustic cavitations is noted

d) Less heat production in spectral Doppler and M-mode than B-mode.
e) Highest attenuation of ultrasound is seen in soft tissue.

75.True regarding definitions

a) Temporal peak intensity refers to the largest intensity at any time during ultrasound exposure.
b) Pulse average intensity is the average over the ultrasound pulse.
c)Temporal average intensity is the average over the entire pulse repetition period.
d)Duty factor is defined as the fraction of time through ultrasound field is on.
e)Dwell time refers to overall duration of the ultrasound exposure to a particular tissue.

76.A transducer with low Q-value (mechanical coefficient) are associated with

a) Light damping.

b) Short ring-down time.
c) Produces shorter pulse.
d) Has lower output of sound.
e) Backing block

77.True regarding transducer

a) Multiple zone focusing mitigate problem of focusing.
b) Like the circular annular array, the beam is focused electronically in only one plane in stepped linear array.
c) Piezoelectronic elements are energized in overlapping groups in stepped linear array.
d) Piezoelectric elements are energized separately in rapid sequence in steered or phase array.
e)Electronic focusing in the elevation plane is made by using a ›1.5 transducer.

78. True regarding ultrasound

a)Higher the angle of incidence (closer to a right angle), greater the amount of reflected sound.
b) The bending of sound as they pass from one medium to another is called refraction.
c)Amount of reflection =(difference in impedance of two tissue/ sum of impedance of two tissue)^{2}X 100.
d)Attenuation refers to total propagation loss including absoption,scattering and reflection.
e)Real structures are imaged in wrong location due to refraction.

79.True regarding annular array mechanical sector transducer

a) Consists of annular array of concentric ring shaped transducer elements.
b) Do not allow focus to be altered(dynamic focusing).
c) Excellent lateral resolution and slice thickness over wide range of depths.
d)Each transducer element in the array operates independent of others.
e)Multiple zone focusing not possible.

80.True regarding ultrasound

contrast agents

a)Improve image quality mainly by increasing the reflections of ultrasound.
b) Based on microbubbles (<4micrometre) or nanoparticles(<1micrometre).
c) Can resonate at ultrasound frequency and at harmonic frequencies.
d)Microbubbles are destroyed by ultrasound of high intensity.
e) Must have low toxicity.

81.True about ultrasound

a) Bone shows lower absorption of ultrasound.
b) In liquid there is high absorption of ultrasound.
c)Longer the relaxation time of substance ,more the absorption ultrasound.
d) The temperature of tissue has no effect over attenuation of ultrasound.
e)Doubling the transducer frequency nearly double the absorption of ultrasound in soft tissue.

82.True regarding ultrasound contrast

a)Intermittent imaging detect strong ,brief, non- linear echo from disrupted bubble.
b)Triggered imaging requires offline processing of stored ultrasound images.
c)Power Doppler imaging is a technique designed to detect the motion of blood or tissue.
d) A low MI ,real- time , nondestructive bubble imaging mode can be used to survey vessels in liver.
e)High MI harmonic power Doppler or pulse inversion can be used for intermittent imaging of liver perfusion with contrast agents.

Answer

ULTRASOUND

1.abcd

Mechanical coefficient = mean frequency /bandwidth.Transducer with high Q-value is good for continuous wave ultrasound. Transducer with low Q-value is god for pulsed ultrasound.

2.abe

Perfluorocarbon nanoparticles stay in blood for many hours after iv .They are slowly taken up by the liver and spleen,improving the image of metastases.

3.abe

A high PRF is chosen for superficial vessel and lower PRF is chosen for deep vessel. The interval between pulses must be long enough for the successive Doppler signal not to overlap. As the range setting is increased ,the PRF is reduced.

4.abe

The thickness of matching layer must be equal to quarter of ultrasound wavelength in the matching layer. Impedance of matching layer must be about mean of the impedances on each side of matching layer (crystal and soft tissue) .

5.acde

Backing block absorbs the backwards travelling waves produced by the back face of the vibrating disc and produce short pulse

6.abcd

7.ad

To avoid aliasing, the Doppler signal must be sampled at least twice in each period. The fastest flow that can be measured with accuracy is the velocity that produces a Doppler shift frequency equal to half the PRF being used. Aliasing does not occurs with continuous wave Doppler.

8. bc

Pulse rate and frequency are different and unrelated The pulse rate refers to number of separate little packets of sound that are sent out each second. Each sonic pulse is short(typically two or three wavelengths.).As the pulse rate increases, the receiving time decreases.At pulse rate of 10000, the thickest part that can be examined is 7.5cm which is satisfactory for ophthalmology.

9. acde

Nearly parallel part of ultrasound beam is known as Fresnel zone. The diverging portion of ultrasound beam is called Fraunhofer zone.

10.bde

Second harmonic is used to produce image. Pulse inversion preserves axial resolution but takes longer time.

11.abcde

12.bcde

Focused transducer improves lateral resolution.

13.abcd

14.abd

The color doesnot indicate velocity or flow direction. Weaker signals can be imaged than in color image.

15. bce

Ultrasound encountering RBCs are scattered in all direction ,referred to as Rayleigh –Tyndall scattering. The intensity of scattered ultrasound wave in Rayleigh- Tyndall scattering increases with the fourth power of the frequency.

16.ade

There is need of compression and remapping of backscattered signal to adapt its the dynamic range to that of the disply.M-mode displays echo amplitude and the position of moving reflectors.

17.ace

Focusing improves the lateral resolution. The shorter focal length produces more divergence.

18.ac

The axial resolution is about half the pulse length. The shorter the pulse length, the better the axial resolution. The axial resolution worsens by omitting backing block and thereby increasing Q.

19.abe

Power Doppler is useful for imaging smaller vessels because weaker signals can be picked up. It is not subject to aliasing .

20.ce

Use of high Q-factor transducer with quarter wave matching is used in CW Doppler.

21.abcde

22.abcde

23.bcd

High frequency ultrasound is more rapidly attenuated and used for superficial structures.

24.ad

Acoustic impedance depends on density and elasticity of material. Fraction of sound energy reflected at the interface between two materials of acoustic impedance z_1 and $z_2 = (z_1-z_2)^2/(z_1+z_2)^2$. Backing block is acoustically matched to the transducer to avoid reflection.

25.abcd

For eye ,10-15MHz transducer is used.

26.cde

The intensity of an ultrasound beam is greatest in the focal region. The time –averaged intensity should nowhere exceed 100 Mw/cm^2

27.acd

CW Doppler does not provide depth information. Gating is used to provide depth information in pulsed Doppler.The depth (often called gate) from which the signal originates is controlled by the length of time after pulse transmission before the transducer is allowed to receive returning signal(the time at which the gate is turned on). The axial length over which the signal originates is determined by the length of time the gate is turned on.
28. cde

Levovist is a dry mixture comprising 99.9% microcrystalline galactose micro particles and 0.1% palmitic acid. It traverses the pulmonary bed.
29.acde

Total reflection of sound energy occurs at any interface with air or gas.
30.abde

Cavitations is less likely with pulse beam.
31..ad

The required time between successive pulses is at least 13 microsecond per cm of range in the sample volume.The maximum Doppler shift frequency that can be detected by a pulsed Doppler system without aliasing is equal to half the pulse repetition frequency(PRF).
32.bcd

Muscle 1.38 x 10^6kg/m^2/s.

Fat 1.70 x 10^6kg/m^2/s.
33.abe

Change of frequency /original(transducer) frequency =2 x (velocity of interface/velocity of sound) x cosine of angle of insonation . Cosine of 90 degree is zero, so no Doppler shift .The Doppler shift frequency is comparatively small.
34.abcde
35.abcde
36.acd

Second generation agent use low solubility gases instead of air and are designed for more backscatter enhancement and to last longer in the blood stream. Useful imaging time while using levovist and echovist(both use air) is considerably less than few minutes .
37.abe
The structures in liver may appear in lung due to double reflection. Negative shadow is due to acoustic enhancement.
38.abcd
39..abcde-
40.bcd

Specular reflectors has large and smooth interface and its display is highly dependent on angle of insonation.
41.abe

Ultrasound cannot be formed into narrow beam as well as light and it is not a electromagnetic wave.
42.abcde

43.ad

Quartz is the naturally occurring material that possess piezoelectric properties. Medical crystal is made to vibrate in thickness mode.

44.ace

Speed of ultrasound increases with increase in temperature. Acoustic impedance does not depend on frequency of ultrasound. Acoustic impedance of tissues differ from each other by few percentage. administered in small quantities. Nonlinear oscillation is the basis of harmonic imaging.

45.abce

The transducer should not be autoclaved . It loses piezoelectric properties above certain temperature (about 350 degree Celsius for PZT),called the Curie temperature.

46.abe

Scattering occurs when sound encounters the structures much smaller than wavelength. Specular reflection follows Snell's rule.(the ratio of the sine's of the incident and refraction angles is equal to the ratio of sound velocities in the two materials.)

47.abe

The thickness of a piezoelectric crystal determines its natural frequency, called resonant frequency. The natural frequency is one that produces internal wavelength that are twice the thickness of the crystal. The frequency that correspond to half of the wavelength thickness is called fundamental resonance frequency.

48.ce

The largest value of the temporal average intensity to be found at any scanned area is known spatial peak temporal intensity. It depend on the machine controls and choice of scanning mode. Pulse bandwidth increases as pulse length decreases.

49.acde

The harmonic response of a ultrasound contrast depend on incident pressure of ultrasound field, frequency ,size distribution of the bubbles and mechanical properties of the bubble capsule.

50.ae

Ultrasound is longitudinal in nature and it can be focused. Its wavelength is sufficiently long for its wave properties(interference and diffraction) to be predominant.

51.acd

The decibel loss in tissue per centimeter is proportional to the frequency. There is little absorption or scatter of ultrasound in water.

52. acde

The transducer should never be autoclaved.

53.abcde
54.ad

The tissue is not completely dark in a typical tissue harmonic image. Because the scanner detect tissue harmonic along with harmonic echo from the bubble. Reverberations are reduced by using tissue harmonic imaging. The tissue harmonic imaging is routine USG modality of choice for visualizing fluid- filled structures.

55.ade

The velocity of ultrasound in a given material is constant, independent of frequency and wavelength. The greater the compressibility (or smaller the elastic modulus), the lower the velocity.

56.abcde

57.ac

High Q- transducer produce sound made up of narrow range of frequencies. It has long ringing time and is unsatisfactory for sonic imaging because returning signal may be lost in the noise of system and long sonic pulse length lowers the depth resolution.

58.abe

Edge effect artifact is due to total internal reflection. In Rayleigh scattering , scattering structures are much smaller than a wavelength.

59.abcde

60.abde

61.abcde

62.ade

Ultrasound takes nearly 7 microsecond to travel each centimeter in average soft tissue. The wavelength of ultrasound (produced by transducer of 3.5MHz) in soft tissue is 0.4mm and in bone is 0.9mm.

63.abc sector scan is used in intracavitary scan and to image heart. Sector scan is easier to manipulate requires a smaller acoustic window and has narrower field near skin.

64.abcde

65.bc

The backing block is incorporated to quench the vibrations and shorten sonic pulse(spatial pulse length=the number of waves x wavelength). The backing block material alter the Q-factor. Impedance of backing block material is similar to that of crystal of transducer crystal.

66.bde

Higher the frequency ,longer the near field length. High frequency unfocussed beams are better collimated than low frequency ones.

67.abcde

68abde

Mechanical sector scanner employs circular transducer.

69.ace

High frequency beam produce longer Fresnel zone. High frequency beam is used for superficial structures.

70.bde

Higher the frequency ,longer the near field length. High frequency unfocussed beams are better collimated than low frequency ones.

71.bde

At natural or resonant frequency, transducer produces a wavelength equal to twice the thickness of the piezoelectric disc and there is largest output of ultrasound. Resonant frequency depend on material of transducer which affect velocity of sound and also on dimensions, particularly on thickness

72.abcde

73.a

Sensitivity depend on the focus position, setting of power output and overall gain control. Sensitivity is greatest close to transit focus. The dynamic range of scanner is measure of the maximum sensitivity that a scanner can achieve. It can be changed.

74.abc

Factors controlling tissue heating are spatial focusing, ultrasound frequency, exposure duration and tissue type. There is more heat production in spectral Doppler and M-mode than B-mode. Highest attenuation of ultrasound is seen in bone.

75.abcde

76.bcde

77.acde

Unlike the circular annular array, the beam is focused electronically in only one plane in stepped linear array.

78.bcde

Higher the angle of incidence (closer to a right angle), lesser the amount of reflected sound.

79.acd

Annular array mechanical sector transducer allow focus to be altered(dynamic focusing) and multiple zone focusing is possible.

80.abcde

81.ce

The attenuation of ultrasound varies with the temperature of the tissues. Higher absorption of ultrasound are noted with higher frequency of ultrasound, higher viscosity of tissue and higher relaxation time of tissue.

82.abcde

CHAPTER 11
MISCELLANEOUS (CONTRAST AGENT, MAMMOGRAPHY , MOLECULAR IMAGING)

1.True regarding iodinated contrast medium

a. tri-iodo benzene ring derivatives with three atoms of iodine at 3,4,6 positions (in monomers)
b. tri-iodo benzene ring derivatives with six atoms of iodine per molecule of the ring anion (in dimers)
c. very hydrophobic , have high lipid solubility, low toxicity,
d. high binding affinities for protein, receptors or membranes
e. have molecular weights less than 2000

2. The 2nd generation non-ionic monomers is /are

a.iohexol
b.iopamidol
c.iopromide
d.ioversol
e. metrizamide

3.True regarding dimers
a. Ioxaglate is only example of ionic dimer
b. Ioxalate is a mixture of the sodium and meglumine salts of a monoacidic double benzene ring
c. Ioxaglate therefore has an iodine:particle ratio of 6:2 or 3:1
d. Ioxalate each benzene ring has three atoms of iodine at C2, 4, 6 positions
e. Ioxalate osmalality about 560

mosmol kg^{-1} water at a concentration of 300 mg I/ml^{-1}

4.True regarding non-ionic dimers
a. Iotrolan (Schering) and iodixanol (Nycomed) are both examples
b. They do not ionize or dissociate in solution.
c. an iodine:particle ratio of 3:1.
d. physiologically isotonic (300 mosmol kg^{-1} water) in solution at 300 mg I/ml^{-1}.
e. Iotrolan widely used has been recently voluntarily withdrawn for intravascular use because of unexpected delayed reactions

5.True regarding ionic monomers (HOCM)

a. sodium or meglumine (N-methyl glucamine) as the non-radio-opaque cation
b. a radio-opaque tri-iodinated fully substituted benzoic acid ring as the anion
c. anions include diatrizoate (Urografin, Hypaque), iothalamate (Conray), ioxithalamate, metrizoate
d. an iodine:particle ratio of 3:2
e. very hypertonic(1600 mosmols kg^{-1} water at 300 mg iodine kg^{-1})compared to physiological osmolality (300 mosmol kg^{-1} water)

6. True regarding adverse reactions of iodinated contrast

a. anaphylactoid reactions are *not dose dependent*

b. non-idiosyncratic reactions relate to the chemical composition, to osmolality and concentration of contrast medium

c. . non-idiosyncratic reactions relate to the volume, speed and multiplicity of the injection.

d. relatively very safe in comparison to other drugs

e. Erythrocyte damage Endothelial damage are due to hyperosmolality

7. True regarding adverse reactions of iodinated contrast

a. severe reactions in about 0.2 per cent after HOCM and about 0.04 per cent following LOCM

b. One death in 40 000 IV injections of HOCM is often quoted as a medium figure.

c. All ADRs are significantly more frequent with HOCM (12.66 per cent) than with LOCM (3.13 per cent)

d. Adrenaline (0.3–0.5 ml, 1/1000 solution [children 0.01 ml kg^{-1} body weight] by deep SC or IM injection

e. Adrenaline is is the main therapeutic agent for severe reactions

8. Adverse predisposing factors for iodinated contrast

a. Patients with a previous ADR to RCM (excluding mild flushing, nausea)

b. Asthmatics

c. Allergic and atopic patients

d. Cardiac patients with decompensation, unstable arrhythmia, recent myocardial infarction

e. Renal patients in failure, diabetic nephropathy, on metformin

9. True regarding iodine

a. The average daily physiological turnover of iodine is 0.0001 g.

b. The total iodine content in the body (mainly in the thyroid) is 0.01 g.

c. The requirement for a 2-, 3- or 4-vessel angiogram (with conventional film-screen photographic recording) may be 70 g iodine

d. Very large amounts of iodine are necessary because of the low sensitivity inherent in conventional photographic film-screen radiography

e. CT scanning and digital subtraction angiography (DSA), are very much more sensitive to minor differences in iodine concentration

10. True regarding extracellular MRI agents

a. Mutagenic and teratogenic effects present

b. avoided in pregnant lady

c. stop breast feeding for 24 hrs prior to administration

d. no prophylaxis before administering extracellular MRI agents

e. *avoid* the administration of non-ionic linear chelates in patients with advanced renal impairment (GFR <30 ml/min) i

11. True regarding non-ionic monomers

a. tri-iodinated non-ionizing compounds

b. provide three atoms of iodine to one osmotically active particle (an iodine:particle ratio of 3:1)

c. less than half of the osmolality of HOCM

d. osmalality about 600 mosmol kg^{-1} water at a concentration of 300 mg I/ml^{-1}

e. Ioxilan, Xenetix are examples

12. True regarding extracellular MRI contrasr agents

a. Generally the recommended dose for clinical use is 0.2 mmol kg^{-1} body weight

b. marked differences in the safety of the various agents

c. The incidence of mild adverse effects is less than 5 per cent.

d. Life-threatening reactions are very rare, with an incidence around 1:100 000

e. high osmolar agents are likely to induce more local damage on extravasation

13. Adverse predisposing factors for iodinated contrast

a. Feeble infants and aged patients

b. Patients with a severe general debility

c. Very nervous, anxious patients

d. sickle cell anemia

e. Thyrotoxic: goitrous patients

14. Drugs useful for treatment of iodinated contrast agent adverse reactions is /are

a. frusemide (Lasix) 20–40 mg IV slowly or IM for pulmonary oedema

b. diazepam and barbiturates for convulsions

c. adrenaline

d. salbutamol

e. aminophylline (*very slowly,* 250–500 mg) intravenously for intense bronchospasm

15. True regarding blood pool contrast agents/persistent vascular agents

a. based on gadolinium compounds or ultrasmall paramagnetic iron oxides (USPIOs)

b. Gadobenate dimeglumine

c. Gadofosveset

d. gadofosveset the short time window .

e. gadofosveset shows contrast uptake in atherosclerotic plaque in late imaging

16. Adverse factors for impairment of renal function by the iodinated contrasts

a. pre-existing renal failure

b. oliguria

c. diabetic nephropathy

d. patients who are not well hydrated

e. patients who are liable to be injected with very high doses of RCM

17. True regarding use of iodinated contrasts

a. The usual recommended dose for IV urography in the normally well-hydrated adult with normal renal function is 15–25 g iodine

b. A maximum of about 70 g of iodine (1 g iodine kg^{-1} body weight in adults) is generally advisable even in patients with good renal function

c. in contrast medium myelography , non-ionic LOCM must be used

d., iophendylate (Myodil, pantopaque) abandoned because it causes severe chronic adhesive arachnoiditis

e. The usual iodine concentration

required for conventional film–screen angiography is about 300 mg I ml⁻¹ contrast medium

18. True regarding adverse effect of iodinated contrast

a. HOCM inhibits thrombosis more than LOCM

b. myelomatosis may develop renal failure after contrast medium injection

c. Patients with phaeochromocytoma may develop a hypertensive crisis during angiography or IV urography

d. Patients with pre-existing renal disease, particularly the renal complications of diabetes mellitus, have an increased risk of an adverse reaction to RCM

e. RCM-related lactic acidosis is extremely rare in diabetics receiving metformin if the patient has normal renal function before RCM

19. True regarding extracellular MR contrast agent

a. paramagnetic compounds

b. reduce only T1 relaxation time

c. increase tissue signal intensity on T1-weighted MR images

d. reduce signal on T2-weighted images.

e. gadolinium diethylene triamine pentacetic acid salt (Gd-DTPA) first agent introduced in clinical practice

20. True regarding pharmacokinetics of most extracellular MRI contrast agents

a. similar to iodinated water-soluble contrast media

b. high molecular mass

c. after IV injection ,rapidly diffuses into the interstitial extravascular space

d. Gd chelates are eliminated through passive glomerular filtration

e. cross the intact specialized vascular blood–brain barrier.

21. True regarding adverse reactions of Extracellular MRI agents

a. Extracellular MRI agents less nephrotoxic than iodinated contrast media in equimolar doses

b. Most of nephrogenic systemc fibrosis complications followed the administration **gadodiamide**

c. least stable molecules are the non ionic linear chelates, and most stable is the ionic cyclic chelate.

d. cross-reaction between extracellular MRI contrast agents and radiographic iodinated contrast media

e. easily removed by haemodialysis or continuous ambulatory peritoneal dialysis

22. Contrast available for MR of liver is/are

a. Magnevist---**Nonspecific extracellular gadolinium chelates**

b. Gd-BOPTA /Gd-EOB-DTPA--**Hepatocyte selective gadolinium chelates**

c. Magafodipir trisodium (MnDPDP)--- Selective uptake by *hepatocytes* and excreted into bile ducts

d. Superparamagnetic iron oxide particles (ferrumoxides 80–150 nm in size)- Selective uptake by *Kupffer* cells

e. Superparamagnetic iron oxide

particles (ferucarbotran 60 nm in size) --Selective uptake by *Kupffer* cells

23. True regading gadobenate dimeglumine (Gd-BOPTA)

a. donot bind to protein

b. eliminated through both the renal and hepatobiliary pathways

c. behaves as a conventional extracellular contrast agent in the first minutes following IV administration

d. behave as liver-specific agent in a later delayed phase (40–120 min after administration)

e. It is taken up specifically by malignant cell

24. True regarding contrast agents

a. gadolinium chelate MR contrast media can be used for measuring varying indices of vascularity

b. microbubbles (ultrasound contrast agents) and technetium (^{99m}Tc)-labelled red blood cells are highly suitable for measuring indices of the blood volume and perfusion in all organs

c. Colloidal agents is selectively taken up into the reticuloendothelial system of the liver and spleen.

d. there is selective uptake of the biliary system (gadolinium ethoxybenzyldiethylenetriaminepentaacetic acid, or Gd-EOB-DTPA) into the biliary system.

e. there is selective uptake of manganese dipyridoxyl diphosphate, or Mn-DPDP by the pancrease.

25. True regarding contrast

a. in general, an increase in iodine density of 1 mg/ml increase

attenuation in a voxel by 10–15HU.

b. MR systems are less sensitive to contrast agents than CT

c. The relative signal change in a region on a T1W can be considered approximately proportional to the local gadolinium concentration when the concentration is high.

d. Microbubbles of USG contrast can be destroyed by the very act of imaging

e. gadolinium ethoxybenzyldiethylenetriaminepentaacetic acid(Gd-EOB-DTPA) is selectively taken by biliary system

26. True regarding advantages of PACS

a. almost instantaneous availability of images in any location

b. simultaneous view of images in different location

c. security of image storage

d. elmination of film stores

e. facility to build teaching files of images

27. True regarding PACS

a. the various imaging devices and associated workstations are linked to the PACS Workflow Manager

b. PACS Workflow Manager refers to the computer and associated software at the heart of PACS

c. PACS Workflow Manager control the flow of images and information

d. DICOM is the standard format of presenting the image file

e. the image file contains only the basic digital data that allow it to be displayed

28. True regarding the PACS

a. The PACS work flow manager can send or retrieve images from the archive

b.the short- term archive is designed for short access on demand

c.For security ,the archive is usually backed up to a seprate archive in a seprate location often at some distance from the hospital

d.A PACS is ineffective if it is not connected to other information systems in the hospital (hospital information system)

e.A PACS broker provides an interface between 'patient administrative system' and the work flow manager

29.True regarding workstations

a.modalty workstations are supplied with the imaging equipment

b.modality workatations can display images from the archive if provided with the appropriate DICOM

c.reporting workstations are generally those used by radiologists

d.the display monitor is calibrated to the DICOM standard to ensure optimum display conditions

e.review workstations has wide range of software

30.True regarding DICOM

a.the service class user role is to invoke an operation

b.the service class provider is to perform the operation

c.CT scan is a user of the storage function of PACS

d.The PACS archive is the provider of storage

e.Modalty push allows the system to store images to PACS

31.Advantages of PACS is /are

a. no loss of or misfiling of image and is always available when needed

b. facilitates the easy comparison of a patient's current and historical imaging examinations

c. image availability all the time

d. Simultaneous multilocation viewing of the same image

e.quicker retrieval of image than hard copy film

32.Advantages of PACS is/are

a.back-up of imaging study

b.numerous post-processing soft-copy manipulations

c.substantial time saving

d.set the stage for teleradiology

e.cheap technology

33.Disadvantages of PACS

a.expensive technology

b. dedicated maintenance programme

c. requirement for new or retrained hospital personnel specializing in computer engineering/information technology

d. no longer equipped to run a film-based service

e. a change of work patterns like the training of the users, maintenance of the system etc

34.True regarding PACS

a. The British Royal College of Radiologists lossy compression for a definitive diagnostic report

b. Lossless compression techniques can currently achieve a maximum compression ratio of 30:1

c. Lossy compression techniques irreversibly compress the image and data are permanently lost,

d. The main requirement for image data compression arises in connection with teleradiology

e. lossy compression algorithm are joint photographic expert group (JPEG) compression, and wavelet compression

35. True regarding perfusion study

a. fractinal vascular volume can be calculated from power Doppler study and tracer kinetics

b. conventional X-ray and MR contrast agents can be used for measurement of direct and indirect indices of permeability
c. global renal function (i.e. GFR) can be determined using serial assays of iodinated contrast agents
d. In microbubble enhancement method, the initial upslope (thick) measures microcirculatory flow speed whilst the asymptote measure is proportional to fractional vascular volume
e. gradient method of perfusion study is affected by venous wash-out

36. Functional indices of vascularity are

a. fractional vascular
b. fractional extravascular volumes
c. perfusion.
d. transit times
e. indices of permeability or contrast clearance

37. True regarding perfusion study

a. concept of chemical microsphere is useful for washed –in studies
b. Semilograthmic plot of time concentration curve is used to calculate perfusion in washed –out studies

c. intracarotid xenon injection for brain perfusion studies is given slowly
d. inhaled inert xenon in CT is given rapidly
e. gradients methods was developed by Miles for functional CT

38. True regarding Washin –in studies of perfusion is/are

a. the agent does not pass through the tissue bed and accumulates progressively in the organ of interest
b. perfusion calculated as the ratio of tissue concentration at equilibrium with the integral of arterial tracer concentration
c. ultrsound contrast agent (microbubbles with diameter > 8microns) may be used
d. chemical microspheres accumulate in the tissue in a manner comparable to intra-arterial microspheres.
e. intra-arterial microspheres use is confined to invasive animal studies

39. True regarding perfusion study (bolus methods)

a. perfusion measured as the ratio of peak parenchymal enhancement to the area under the arterial time–enhancement curve
b. perfusion calculated from the ratio of the peak gradient of the tissue time–concentration curve to the peak height of the arterial curve(gradient method)
c. gradient method applicable to measurement of liver blood flow
d. One of the approach is measurements of mean transit time (MTT) for a tracer to pass from

inflow to outflow

E. Microbubbles offer a particularly appealing and elegant method of measuring true vascular transit times

40. True regarding molecular imaging

a. Direct molecular imaging involves direct interaction between the imaging probe and the molecular target (e.g. a specific enzyme or receptor).

b. Surrogate molecular imaging reflects the downstream physiological effects of one or more molecular or genetic processes.

c. Indirect molecular imaging strategies typically involving reporter gene

d. Differences in gene expression at different disease sites in the same patient and changing expression over is appreciated through molecular imaging

e. molecular imaging can assess molecular and genetic processes in the target tissue and other organs simultaneously.

41. True regarding reporter gene imaging

a. The reporter gene is incorporated into the nuclear RNA of the target cells by transfection (e.g. viral vector

b. The activated reporter gene is transcribed into the corresponding messenger ribonucleic acid (mRNA)

c. messenger RNA (mRNA) is translated to the reporter protein

d. a reporter substrate is admninistered

e. The reporter substrate interacts with the reporter protein to produce

an imaging signal (e.g. gamma ray, paramagnetic effect).

42.. True regarding reporter gene –substrate combination

a. the herpes simplex virus type 1 thymidine kinase (HSV1-TK) and fluoro-deoxy-arabinofuranosyl-iodouracil or FIAU

b. genes encoding for a modified human transferrin receptor and supraparamagnetic iron compounds

c. β-galactosidase and gadolinium contrast agent (EgadMe)

d. the herpes simplex virus type 1 thymidine kinase (HSV1-TK) and (EgadMe)

e. the herpes simplex virus type 1 thymidine kinase (HSV1-TK) and gadolinium contrast agent (EgadMe)

43. True regarding molecular imaging

a. increased FDG uptake in a variety of tumours and in hypoxic tissue

b. fluorodeoxyglucose (FDG) PET and ^{99m}Tc methoxyisobutylisonitrile (MIBI) scintigraphy are example of indirect molecular imaging

c. FDG interacts in*directly* with Glut-1 glucose transporters

d. ^{99m}Tc-MIBI interacts *directly* with a p-glycoprotein (pgp) that produces multidrug resistance in tumours

e. rapid elimination of MIBI in delayed image imply drug resistance

44. True regarding potential of use of molecular imaging

a. development of gene therapies

b. development of drugs that have specific molecular targets (e.g. an anticancer drug that aims to block VEGF activity).

c. used in drug trials to identify subpopulations of patients enriched for response, increasing the probability of demonstrating drug efficacy

d. The use of molecular imaging as a response marker

e. to select patients for specific therapy and to assess therapeutic response

45.True regarding hypoxia – inducible factor(HIF-1)

a.increased in hypoxia

b.decreased in oncogene mutations(von Hippel–Lindau (VHL) gene or mutations in the p53 suppressor gene)

c.a translation factor

d.up regulate molecule like nitric oxide,VEGF

e.down regulate GLUT-1 and MDR_p-G_p

46.True regading terminology

a. DICOM stands for **di**gital **co**mmunication in **me**dicine

b.DICOM refers to a worldwide multipart standard to which all modern imaging equipment

c.HL7 stands for **h**ealth **l**evel **7** and refers to a worldwide standard for data information systems such as HIS and RIS

d. HL7 is a less rigorous standard than DICOM

e. IHE stands for **i**ntegrating the **h**ealth care **e**nterprise and is not a standard, but a comprehensive workflow descriptor of how processes, such as reporting, for example, are achieved in imaging

ANSWER

MISCELLANEOUS (CONTRAST AGENT,MAMMOGRAPHY, MOLECULAR IMAGING)

1.be---- iodinated contrast medium is tri-iodo benzene ring derivatives with three atoms of iodine at 2,4,6 positions (in monomers) and with six atoms of iodine per molecule of the ring anion (in dimers).They are very hydrophilic, have low lipid solubility, low toxicity, low binding affinities for protein, receptors or membranes,have molecular weights less than 2000.(CHAPTER 2 ,Adam: Grainger)

2. abcd---- Almén introduced the concept of non-ionic (and therefore low osmolar) contrast media in 1969 with metrizamide.(CHAPTER 2 ,Adam: Grainger)

3.abcde---.(CHAPTER 2 ,Adam: Grainger)

4.abd---- Iotrolan (Schering) and iodixanol (Nycomed) are both examples of non ionic dimers has an iodine:particle ratio of 3:1.Iotrolan widely used has been recently voluntarily withdrawn for intravascular use because of unexpected delayed reactions(more in Japanese).
.(CHAPTER 2 ,Adam: Grainger)

5.abcde----(CHAPTER 2 ,Adam: Grainger)

6.abcde---- (CHAPTER 2 ,Adam: Grainger)

7.abcde-----(CHAPTER 2 ,Adam: Grainger)

8.abcde---- (CHAPTER 2 ,Adam: Grainger)

9.abcde----(CHAPTER 2 ,Adam: Grainger)

10. de---Extracellular MRI agents has no mutagenic and teratogenic effects present,so may be given in avoided in pregnant lady and there is no need to stop breast feeding for 24 hrs prior to administration.(CHAPTER 2 ,Adam: Grainger)

11.abcde---- .(CHAPTER 2 ,Adam: Grainger)

12.cde----- Generally the recommended dose of extracellular MRI contrasr agents for clinical use is 0.1 mmol kg^{-1} body weight .There is no differences in the safety of the various agents. .(CHAPTER 2 ,Adam: Grainger)

13. abcde----.(CHAPTER 2 ,Adam: Grainger)

14.abcde------(CHAPTER 2 ,Adam: Grainger)

15.abce----Gadofosveset shows the very prolonged time window T ½ of 28 min (compared to 90s for Gad-DTPA) and also shows contrast uptake in atherosclerotic plaque in late imaging. .(CHAPTER 2 ,Adam: Grainger)

16. abcde-----(CHAPTER 2 ,Adam: Grainger)

17.abcde------.(CHAPTER 2 ,Adam: Grainger)

18.abcde------.(CHAPTER 2 ,Adam: Grainger)

19.ace-----extracellular MR contrast agent are paramagnetic compounds which reduce T1 and T2 relaxation time and have almost no effect on T2-weighted images. .(CHAPTER 2 ,Adam: Grainger)

20.acd----- Pharmacokinetics of of most extracellular MRI contrast agents is similar to iodinated water-soluble contrast media,has low molecular mass and do not cross the intact specialized vascular blood–brain barrier. (CHAPTER 2 ,Adam: Grainger)

21.bce---- Extracellular MRI agents are more nephrotoxic than iodinated contrast media in equimolar doses.There is no cross-reaction between extracellular MRI contrast agents and radiographic iodinated contrast media. .(CHAPTER 2 ,Adam: Grainger)

22. abcde------.(CHAPTER 2 ,Adam: Grainger)

23.bcd----Gadobenate dimeglumine (Gd-BOPTA) has capacity for weak and transient protein binding.It is taken up specifically by normal hepatocytes. .(CHAPTER 2 ,Adam: Grainger)

24.abcde-----.(CHAPTER 2 ,Adam: Grainger)

25.de---- In general, an increase in iodine density of 1 mg/ml increase attenuation in a voxel by 25–30HU.MR systems are more sensitive to contrast agents than CT. The relative signal change in a region on a T1W can be considered approximately proportional to the local gadolinium concentration when the concentration is low. (CHAPTER 2 ,Adam: Grainger)

26.abcde---(page no.88/Farr).

27.abcd----- The image file contains not only the basic digital data that allow it to be displayed ,but it also contains essential information including the imaging modality,annotations,display preferences,the patients name and other identifying data. ---(page no.88/Farr).

28.acde---- In The PACS the short-term archive is designed for rapid access on demand. (page no.89/Farr).

29.abcd--- Review workstations has limited imaging software.Primary reporting from review workstations should be done with caution(page no.88/Farr).

30.abcde------(page no.88/Farr).

31.abcde-----(CHAPTER 1 ,Adam: Grainger .)

32.abcde-------(CHAPTER 1 ,Adam: Grainger)

33.abcde----(CHAPTER 1 ,Adam: Grainger)

34.de---The British Royal College of Radiologists lossless compression for a definitive diagnostic report.Lossless compression techniques can currently achieve a maximum compression ratio of 3:1. As the name implies, lossless compression reversibly compresses the data so that no data are permanently lost from the image. (CHAPTER 1 ,Adam: Grainger)

35.abcde---(CHAPTER 1 ,Adam: Grainger)

36.abcde----(CHAPTER 1 ,Adam: Grainger)

37.abcde----(CHAPTER 1 ,Adam: Grainger)

38.abcde----(CHAPTER 1 ,Adam: Grainger)

39.abcde----(CHAPTER 1 ,Adam: Grainger)

40.abcde-----(CHAPTER 1 ,Adam: Grainger)

41.abcde----(CHAPTER 1 ,Adam: Grainger)

42.abcde-----(CHAPTER 1 ,Adam: Grainger)

43.abcde-----(CHAPTER 1 ,Adam: Grainger)

44 abcde-----(CHAPTER 1 ,Adam: Grainger)

45 abcde-----(CHAPTER 1 ,Adam: Grainger)

46.ad---- Hypoxia –inducible factor(HIF-1) is incresed in oncogene mutations(von Hippel–Lindau (VHL) gene or mutations in the p53 suppressor gene),it is a transcription factor and up-regulate GLUT-1 and MDR_p-G_p.(CHAPTER 1 ,Adam: Grainger)

47.abcde----(CHAPTER 1 ,Adam: Grainger)

END

SUGGESTED REFERENCE BOOKS

1. Christensen's Physics of Diagnostic radiology.Third edition by Curry   and Dowdy.Published by Lippincott and Raven.

2. Physics for Diagnostic Radiology,second edition by P PDendy and B Heaton

3. Farr'sPhysics for medical imaging.Secon edition byPenelopeAllisy Roberts and Jerry Williams.Published by Saunders.

4. Clinical magnetic resonance imaging.Third edition ,edited by Edelman,Hesselink,Zlatkin an Crues III .Published   saunders.

5. Adam: Grainger & Allison's Diagnostic Radiology, 5th ed.

ABOUT THE AUTHOR

A consultant radiologist ,Dr Nagendra kumar sinha has passed MBBS from Patna Medical College and Hospital ,Patna (Bihar ,India) and got his MD (Radiodiagnosis) degree from Assam medical College and Hospital,Dibrugarh(Assam,India).He has worked as DM (Neuroradiology) resident at AIIMS,New Delhi (India).

He administers Nagendra's Radiology Blog (http://nagendraradiology.blogspot.com/) and Path To Sucess blog (http://nagendraway.blogspot.com/).He has keen interest in personality development and matters of spritualism.

He is the author of two books --FRCR MCQs Physics MRI and USG

(Amazon.com) and MCQs in Radiology(Amazon.com). He remains actively involved in different different CMEs and conferences .

Printed in Great Britain
by Amazon